The Complete Dash Diet Cookbook for Beginners

600 Fresh and Delicious Recipes to Lose Weight Fast

By Joseph Baker

Copyright © Joseph Baker

All rights reserved.

No part of this guide may be reproduced in any form without permission in writing from the publisher except in the case of brief quotations embodied in critical articles or reviews.

Legal & Disclaimer

The information contained in this book and its contents is not designed to replace or take the place of any form of medical or professional advice; and is not meant to replace the need for independent medical, financial, legal or other professional advice or services, as may be required. The content and information in this book has been provided for educational and entertainment purposes only.

The content and information contained in this book has been compiled from sources deemed reliable, and it is accurate to the best of the Author's knowledge, information and belief. However, the Author cannot guarantee its accuracy and validity and cannot be held liable for any errors and/or omissions. Further, changes are periodically made to this book as and when needed. Where appropriate and/or necessary, you must consult a professional (including but not limited to your doctor, attorney, financial advisor or such other professional advisor) before using any of the suggested remedies, techniques, or information in this book.

You agree that by continuing to read this book, where appropriate and/or necessary, you shall consult a professional (including but not limited to your doctor, attorney, or financial advisor or such other advisor as needed) before using any of the suggested remedies, techniques, or information in this book.

Table of Contents

Introduction 1	Peanut Butter with Chia Seeds Overnight Oats..21
Chapter 1 DASH Diet 101 2	Sunday Morning Waffles................................22
Why the DASH Diet Works................................ 3	Oat Smoothie.. 22
DASH Diet Benefits... 3	Saturday Morning Pancakes.......................... 22
DASH Diet Health Plan..................................... 5	Breakfast Banana Split..................................23
Steps Towards Transitioning to the DASH Diet.. 5	Multigrain Hot Cereal................................... 23
The do's and don'ts of Food............................. 6	Quinoa Porridge... 23
Creating a Meal Plan.. 8	French Toasts Casserole................................ 24
Utensils and Cookware.................................... 8	Delicious Omelet.. 24
Chapter 2 Breakfast Recipes.........................9	Chicken Breakfast Burrito............................. 24
Sweet Potatoes with Coconut Flakes................9	Breakfast Sausage Crepe Filling.....................25
Flaxseed & Banana Smoothie...........................9	Banana Bread... 25
Fruity Tofu Smoothie..9	Spinach Muffins..25
French Toast with Applesauce........................10	Chia Seeds Breakfast Mix............................. 26
Banana-Peanut Butter 'n Greens Smoothie........ 10	Breakfast Fruits Bowls...................................26
Baking Powder Biscuits..................................10	Easy Omelet Waffles.................................... 26
Oatmeal Banana Pancakes with Walnuts........... 11	Pesto Omelet.. 26
Creamy Oats, Greens & Blueberry Smoothie.... 11	Strawberry Sandwich................................... 27
Banana & Cinnamon Oatmeal........................ 11	Irish Brown Bread...27
Bagels Made Healthy..................................... 11	Fresh Fruit Crunch.. 27
Cereal with Cranberry-Orange Twist............... 12	Apple and Quinoa Breakfast Bake................. 28
No Cook Overnight Oats................................ 12	Banana and Pear Breakfast Salad.................. 28
Avocado Cup with Egg.................................. 12	Apple Cinnamon Crisp................................. 28
Mediterranean Toast...................................... 13	Peanut Butter & Blueberry Parfait.................29
Instant Banana Oatmeal................................. 13	Quinoa Quiche... 29
Almond Butter-Banana Smoothie.................... 13	Sweet Rosemary Oats................................... 29
Brown Sugar Cinnamon Oatmeal.................... 13	Egg Parsley Omelet...................................... 29
Buckwheat Pancakes with Vanilla Almond Milk14	Quinoa Breakfast Bars.................................. 30
Tomato Bruschetta with Basil......................... 14	Granola Breakfast Pops................................ 30
Sweet Corn Muffins....................................... 14	Cinnamon Breakfast Quinoa..........................30
Scrambled Eggs with Mushrooms and Spinach. 15	Cinnamon Walnut Breakfast Parfait............... 31
Chia and Oat Breakfast Bran.......................... 15	Breakfast Taco... 31
Faux Breakfast Hash Brown Cups................... 15	Egg Spinach Breakfast Muffins......................31
Maple Mocha Frappe..................................... 16	Whole Grain Toast with Fruited Ricotta Spread 32
Breakfast Oatmeal in Slow Cooker................. 16	Cherries Oatmeal.. 32
Apple Cinnamon Overnight Oats.................... 16	Strawberry Chia Breakfast Pudding................32
Hot Honey Porridge....................................... 17	Banana Nutty Oats.. 32
French Toast with Cinnamon Vanilla................17	Breakfast Apple and Raisin Oatmeal..............33
Breakfast Grains and Fruits............................ 17	Fast Punch... 33
Eggs with Cheese.. 18	Chocolate Covered Banana Quinoa...............33
Hearty Orange Peach Smoothie...................... 18	**Chapter 3 Vegetarian and Vegan**......................34
Cheddar & Kale Frittata................................. 18	Baked Potatoes and "BBQ" Lentils................34
Spinach Mushroom Omelette......................... 19	Orange Juice Smoothie................................. 34
Spinach 'n Tomato Egg Scramble................... 19	Superb Lemon Roasted Artichokes................ 34
Mango and Coconut Oatmeal......................... 19	Chocolate Aquafaba Mousse......................... 35
Hearty Green Smoothie................................. 20	Hearty Baby Carrots..................................... 35
Quick Turmeric Oatmeal................................ 20	Sensitive Steamed Artichokes........................ 36
Berry Bowl... 20	Minted Peas Feta Rice.................................. 36
Delicious Flaxseed Banana Porridge............... 21	Rhubarb and Strawberry Compote................. 36
Greens and Ginger Smoothie.......................... 21	Zucchini Cakes..37

Fresh Fruit Smoothie 37
Popovers 37
Broccoli, Garlic, and Rigatoni 38
Vegan Rice Pudding 38
Cinnamon-scented Quinoa 38
Green Vegetable Smoothie 39
Garlic Lovers Hummus 39
Spinach and Kale Mix 39
Apples and Cabbage Mix 39
Thyme Mushrooms 40
Rosemary Endives 40
Roasted Beets 40
Minty Tomatoes and Corn 40
Pesto Green Beans 41
Sage Carrots 41
Dates and Cabbage Sauté 41
Baked Squash Mix 41
Kale Sauté 42
Lemony Endives 42
Garlic Mushrooms and Corn 42
Cilantro Broccoli 43
Paprika Carrots 43
Mashed Cauliflower 43
Spinach Spread 43
Mustard Greens Sauté 44
Basil Turnips Mix 44
Baked Mushrooms 44
Celery and Kale Mix 45
Spicy Avocado 45
Cauliflower Risotto 45
Kale Dip 45
Dill Cabbage 46
Curried Cauliflower Steaks with Red Rice ... 46

Chapter 4 Poultry 47
Parmesan and Chicken Spaghetti Squash ... 47
Apricot Chicken 47
Oven-fried Chicken Breasts 47
Rosemary Roasted Chicken 48
Artichoke and Spinach Chicken 48
Pumpkin and Black Beans Chicken 48
Chicken Thighs and Apples Mix 49
Thai Chicken Thighs 49
Falling "Off" The Bone Chicken 49
Feisty Chicken Porridge 50
The Ultimate Faux-Tisserie Chicken 50
Oregano Chicken Thighs 50
Pesto Chicken Breasts with Summer Squash ... 51
Chicken, Tomato and Green Beans 51
Chicken Tortillas 51
Slow-roast Chicken with Homemade Gravy ... 52
Balsamic Chicken Mix 52
Turkey Pinwheels 53
Salsa Chicken 53
Cajun Chicken and Rice 53
Chicken, Scallions and Carrot Mix 54
Chicken and Bell Peppers 54
Chicken Cranberry Meal 54
Hot Chicken Mix 55
Asian Glazed Chicken 55
Heavenly Garlic Chicken and Sprouts 55
Italian Chicken Wings 56
Smoked Chicken and Apple Mix 56
Creamy Chicken 56
Chicken and Veggies 57
Hidden Valley Chicken Drummies 57
Lemon-parsley Chicken Breast 57
Chicken and Brussels Sprouts 58
Chicken Divan 58
Spicy Pulled Chicken Wraps 58
Apricot Chicken Wings 59
Chicken and Broccoli 59
Balsamic Roast Chicken 59
Chicken, Bell Pepper & Spinach Frittata 60
Hot Chicken Wings 60
Balsamic Chicken and Beans 60
Butter Chicken 61
Five-Spice Roasted Duck Breasts 61
Chicken and Radish Mix 61
Chicken with Broccoli 62
Chicken, Pasta and Snow Peas 62
Chicken with Ginger Artichokes 62
Roast Chicken Dal 63
Stovetop Barbecued Chicken Bites 63
Champion Chicken Pockets 63
Peach Chicken Treat 64
Baked Chicken Pesto 64
Coconut-Crusted Lime Chicken 64
Chicken and Avocado Bake 65
Balsamic Chicken over Greens 65
Chicken Chopstick 65
Balsamic Turkey and Peach Mix 66
Chicken and Asparagus Mix 66
Chicken and Dill Green Beans Mix 66
Turkey with Beans and Olives 67
Parmesan Turkey 67
Chicken and Beets Mix 67
Turkey and Bok Choy 67
Creamy Chicken and Shrimp Mix 68
Allspice Chicken Wings 68
Cheddar Turkey Mix 68
Turkey with Celery Salad 69
Lemony Leek and Chicken 69
Chicken and Corn 69
Chicken and Snow Peas 69
Turkey and Berries 70
Balsamic Baked Turkey 70

Turkey with Spiced Greens.................................70
Chapter 5 Fish and Seafood............................. 71
   Mighty Garlic and Butter Sword Fish................71
   Thai Coconut Tilapia and Rice........................71
   Supreme Cooked Lobster................................71
   Tilapia with Parsley..72
   Pressure Cooker Crab Legs............................72
   Salmon and Broccoli Medley...........................72
   Tilapia with Lemon Garlic Sauce.....................73
   Easy Coconut Shrimp......................................73
   Shrimp Quesadillas..73
   The OG Tuna Sandwich..................................74
   Easy To Understand Mussels..........................74
   Chili-Rubbed Tilapia with Asparagus & Lemon 74
   Parmesan-Crusted Fish...................................75
   Tuna Melt Delight..75
   Uber-Cool Salmon Steaks...............................75
   Crustless Crab "Quiche".................................76
   Godly Garlic Butter Salmon Asparagus............76
   Steamed Blue Crabs.......................................77
   Capelin Balls..77
   Southwestern Salmon....................................77
   Pressure Cooker Salmon Steaks......................78
   Salmon and Horseradish Sauce......................78
   Simple Grilled Tilapia......................................78
   Crunchy Topped Fish with Potato Sticks..........79
   Easy Sautéed Fish Fillets................................79
   Tasty Halibut and Cherry Tomatoes.................79
   Salmon and Cauliflower Mix...........................80
   Creamy Salmon and Asparagus Mix.................80
   Salmon in Dill Sauce......................................80
   Easy Salmon and Brussels Sprouts..................81
   Shrimp Lo Mein..81
   Salmon and Potatoes Mix...............................81
   Smoked Salmon and Radishes.......................82
   Parmesan Baked Fish.....................................82
   Shrimp and Mango Mix..................................82
   Roasted Hake...82
   Coconut Cream Shrimp..................................83
   Simple Cinnamon Salmon..............................83
   Lemon-Herb Grilled Fish.................................83
   Scallops and Strawberry Mix...........................84
   Cod Peas Relish...84
   Chipotle Spiced Shrimp..................................84
   Baked Haddock...85
   Basil Tilapia..85
   Lemony Mussels..85
   Hot Tuna Steak..86
   Spicy Baked Fish..86
   Marinated Fish Steaks....................................86
   Baked Tomato Hake.......................................87
   Cheesy Tuna Pasta...87
   Herb-Coated Baked Cod with Honey...............87

Tender Salmon in Mustard Sauce......................88
Broiled White Sea Bass....................................88
Steamed Fish Balls..88
Lemony & Creamy Tilapia................................89
Smoked Trout Spread.....................................89
Broiled Sea Bass...89
Spicy Cod...89
Lemon Salmon with Kaffir Lime.......................90
Heartfelt Tuna Melt...90
Crab Salad...90
Minty Cod Mix..91
Salmon and Dill Capers...................................91
Creamy Sea Bass Mix.....................................91
Tuna and Shallots...91
Paprika Tuna..92
Ginger Sea Bass Mix......................................92
Parmesan Cod Mix...92
Chapter 6 Beef, Pork and Lamb....................... 93
   Authentic Pepper Steak..................................93
   Lamb Chops with Rosemary...........................93
   Cane Wrapped Around In Prosciutto...............93
   Beef Veggie Pot Meal.....................................94
   Braised Beef Shanks......................................94
   Beef Heart...94
   Beef with Mushrooms....................................94
   Lemony Braised Beef Roast............................95
   Grilled Fennel-Cumin Lamb Chops..................95
   Jerk Beef and Plantain Kabobs........................95
   Beef Pot...96
   Beef with Cucumber Raita..............................96
   Bistro Beef Tenderloin....................................96
   The Surprising No "Noodle" Lasagna...............97
   Lamb Chops with Kale....................................97
   Thyme Beef and Potatoes Mix........................98
   Lamb and Bok Choy Pan................................98
   Simple Veal Chops...98
   Beef & Vegetable Stir-fry................................99
   Beef and Barley Farmers Soup.......................99
   Simple Pork and Capers.................................99
   A "Boney" Pork Chop....................................100
   Roast and Mushrooms..................................100
   Easy Pork Chops...100
   Pork and Celery Mix......................................101
   Pork and Dates Sauce...................................101
   Pork Roast and Cranberry Roast....................101
   Pork and Roasted Tomatoes Mix....................102
   Provence Pork Medallions.............................102
   Garlic Pork Shoulder.....................................102
   Pork Patties..103
   Tarragon Pork Steak.....................................103
   Pork Meatballs..103
   Winter Pork Roast...104
   Pork and Cabbage Salad...............................104

Mustard Pork Chops.................................... 104
Pork Chops and Apples............................. 105
Pork Belly and Apple Sauce..................... 105
Pork and Fennel Mix..................................105
Pork Chop Casserole................................. 106
Pork and Red Peppers Mix........................ 106
Black Currant Jam Pork Chops................ 106
Pork and Cabbage Casserole.................... 107
Coconut Pork Chops.................................. 107
Curried Pork and Cabbage........................ 107
Pork with Apple... 108
Nutmeg Pork Chops................................... 108
Butter and Dill Pork Chops.......................109
Paprika Pork with Carrots......................... 109
Pork and Greens Mix................................. 109
Sage Pork Chops.. 110
Pork with Avocados................................... 110
Pork with Chickpeas.................................. 110
Pork and Mint Corn................................... 111
Pork Chops and Snow Peas....................... 111
Pork and Leeks Soup................................. 111
Pork with Peaches Mix.............................. 112
Allspice Pork Chops and Olives............... 112
Pork Meatballs... 112
Pork and Endives....................................... 113
Pork with Brussels Sprouts....................... 113
Pork with Sprouts and Capers................... 113
Pork with Beets.. 114
Pork and Green Onions Mix..................... 114
Pork with Herbs de Provence.................... 114
Pork and Carrots Soup............................... 115
Chili Pork... 115

Chapter 7 Side Dishes and Appetizers.............. 116
Cauliflower and Potato Mash.................... 116
Grilled Asparagus...................................... 116
Garlic Steamed Squash.............................. 116
Satisfying Corn Cob...................................117
Devilled Eggs...117
Borders Apart Mexican Cauliflower Rice........ 117
Egg and Bean Medley................................ 118
Cheddar and Apple Panini Sandwich....... 118
Roasted Carrots.. 118
Fancy Red and White Sprouts.................. 119
Garlic and Chive "Mash"...........................119
Crashing Asparagus Risotto with Microstock..119
Turkey and Melted Cheese Sandwich...... 120
Garlic and Broccoli Mismash.................... 120
Crunchy Creamy Mashed Sweet Potatoes........120
Ultimate Roast Potatoes............................ 121
Personal and Intimate Soy Milk............... 121
Extremely Crazy Egg Devils..................... 122
Green Pea purée... 122
Herbed Green Beans.................................. 122

Easy Lemon Roasted Radishes........................122
Green Beans with Nuts...................................123
Beets stewed with Apples..............................123
Cabbage Quiche..123
Baked Tomatoes... 124
Cabbage Rolls Stuffed with Dried Apricots.....124
Rice and Chicken Stuffed Tomatoes............. 124
Squash Pancakes.. 125
Avocado Dip... 125
Stuffed Turnips.. 125
Apples Stuffed with Quark............................ 125
Baked Pumpkin Oatmeal............................... 126
Meringue Cookies.. 126
Rose Hip Jelly.. 126
Easy Broccoli and Penne............................... 127
Berry Soufflé..127
White Sponge Cake....................................... 127
Roasted Asparagus... 128
Rigatoni with Broccoli.................................. 128
Rutabaga Puree.. 128
Pan Seared Acorn Squash and Pecans.............. 129
Shaved Brussels Sprouts with Walnuts........ 129
Honey Mustard Chicken Fillets.................... 129
Grilled Pesto Shrimps................................... 130
Rosemary Potato Shells................................ 130
Basil Tomato Crostini................................... 130
Cranberry Spritzer..131
Butternut Squash Fries...................................131

Chapter 8 Snacks and Desserts........................ 132
Healthy Chocolate Avocado Pudding............132
Date-a-Peanut Snack Bars............................. 132
Lemony Chickpeas Dip................................. 132
Baked Stuffed Apples.................................... 133
Basmati Rice Pudding with Oranges............ 133
Berry Yogurt Popsicles................................. 133
Chili Nuts... 134
Apples and Cream Shake.............................. 134
Lemony Kale Popcorn................................... 134
Perfect Hard-Boiled Eggs............................. 135
Chickpeas and Pepper Hummus................... 135
Tortilla Chips... 135
Almond Rice Pudding....................................135
Sweet Potatoes and Apples Mix................... 136
Sautéed Bananas with Orange Sauce........... 136
Caramelized Blood Oranges with Ginger Cream 136
Grilled Minted Watermelon.......................... 137
Caramelized Apricot Pots............................. 137
Melon Mojito Granita................................... 137
Mocha Pops.. 138
Rhubarb Pie.. 138
Berry No Bake Bars...................................... 138
Tropical Fruit Napoleon................................ 139
Ginger Peach Pie..139

Mocha Ricotta Cream 140
Fresh Parfait 140
Easy Fudge 140
Fruit Skewers 140
Easy Pomegranate Mix 141
Berries Mix 141
Broccoli Bites 141
Coconut Mousse 141
Blueberry Cream 142
Lemon Apple Mix 142
Minty Rhubarb 142
Nigella Mango Sweet Mix 142
Blueberry Compote 143
Lentils and Dates Brownies 143
Blueberry Curd 143
Almond Peach Mix 144
Coconut Cream 144
Cinnamon Apples 144
Green Tea Cream 144
Coconut Figs 145
Cocoa Banana Dessert Smoothie 145
Chocolate Pomegranate Fudge 145
Cashew Nut Cuppas 145
Cheese Stuffed Apples 146
Green Apple Bowls 146
Peach Dip 146
Pecan Granola 147
Walnut Green Beans 147
Banana Sashimi 147
Maple Malt 147
Parmesan Roasted Chickpeas 148
Apricot Nibbles 148
All Dressed Crispy Potato Skins 148
Delightful Coconut Shrimp 149
Creamy Peanuts with Apples 149

Chapter 9 Stews and Soups 150
Vegetarian Split Pea Soup in a Crock Pot 150
Rhubarb Stew 150
Tofu Soup 150
Easy Beef Stew 151
Zucchini-Basil Soup 151
Black Bean Soup 151
Chicken and Dill Soup 152
Cherry Stew 152
Sirloin Carrot Soup 152
Easy Wonton Soup 153
Sweet Potato Soup 153
Omnipotent Organic Chicken Thigh Soup 153
Minty Grapefruit Stew 154
Apple Butternut Soup 154
Beef Soup 154
Strawberry Soup a La Kiev 154
Summer Strawberry Stew 155

Peach Stew 155
Eggplant Soup 155
Blueberry Stew 155
Leek and Chicken Soup 156
Courgette, Pea & Pesto Soup 156
Watermelon Stew 156
Apricots Stew 156
Grapes Stew 157
Zucchini Cream Soup 157
Beef Prune Stew 157

Chapter 10 Salads and Sauces 158
New Potato Salad 158
Potato & Octopus Salad 158
Balsamic Beet Salad 158
Mango Tango Salad 159
Terrific Tortellini Salad 159
Squash Garden Salad 159
Beet, Prune and Walnut Salad 160
Steamed Saucy Garlic Greens 160
Scoop-It-Up Chicken Salad 160
Daikon Radish Salad 161
Boiled Carrot Salad with Green Peas ... 161
Faux Soy Sauce 161
Citrus Shrimp Salad 161
Calamari Salad 162
Shrimp and Asparagus Salad 162
Carrot and Walnut Salad 162
Pickled Onion Salad 162
Chicken Raisin Salad 163
Pickled Grape Salad with Pear, Taleggio and Walnuts 163
Mango Salad 163
Fresh Fruit Salad 164
Dried Apricot Sauce 164
Tomato, Cucumber, and Basil Salad 164
Strawberries and Avocado Salad 165
Kelp Salad 165
Chicken Celery Salad 165
Garlic Potato Salad 165
Spring Salad 166
Appetizing Cucumber Salad 166
Pumpkin Salad 166
Tuna Caprese Salad 167
Cabbage and Carrot Salad 167
Warm Asparagus Salad with Oranges ... 167
Chicken in Orange Sauce 168
Sweet Jicama Salad 168
Heart Healthy Chicken Salad 168
Cashews and Blueberries Salad 169
Radish Salad 169
Tarragon Tomatoes 169

Appendix 30 Day Meal Plan 170
Conclusion 173

Introduction

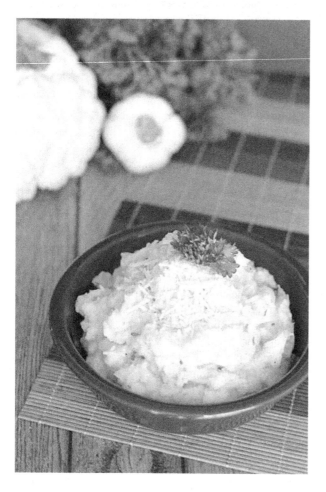

Are you aware of the Dash Diet?
Do you understand the benefits accrued to the diet?
Are you suffering from blood pressure?
Do you wish to reduce the risks of blood pressure?
Do you look forward to losing the extra pounds and lead a healthy lifestyle?
Do you yearn to enjoy delicious foods to increase longevity?

Most people consider the DASH Diet as a dietary recipe for dealing with high blood pressure; however, recent studies have actually shown that there are more benefits lurking within this diet than blood pressure treatment.

The DASH diet is able to lower blood pressure and speed up fat burning in the body because it lowers the amount of LDL (bad cholesterol in the body) and then speeds up metabolism. The combined effect of these is that the body will gradually replace excess fat with lean muscle.

The DASH diet is all about substituting certain nutrients in regular day-to-day diets, for instance, reducing sodium and increasing the uptake of potassium, magnesium, and calcium has been found to lower blood pressure, and increase metabolism while providing essential minerals for the optimal working of body cells.

The typical DASH diet comes with numerous low glycemic foods that ensure lower blood sugar, which in turn reduces insulin intolerance in the body; therefore, such a diet can play a critical role in reversing diseases such as diabetes.

This book deals with the basics of the DASH diet and the health plan to adopt. It will also deal with how to get started with the diet. It is a boon for people who are trying to get their blood pressure under control.

Once you learn about the diet, I have collated a wide array of recipes that will make sure you have a good variety for you and your family when you follow the DASH diet.

Are you ready? Get a copy of this book and keep on reading. This book will give you more answers to the above questions...

Chapter 1 DASH Diet 101

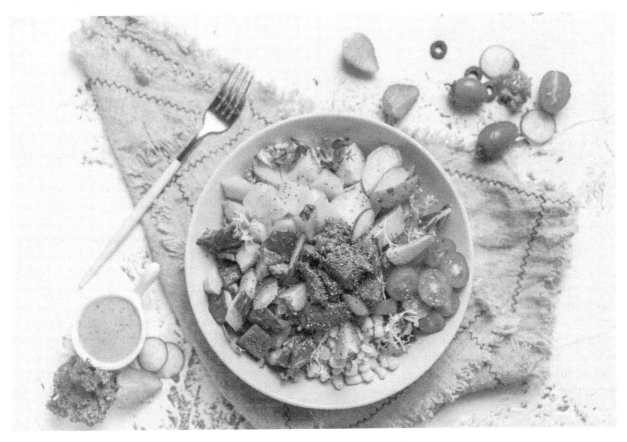

I'm sure you've been through diets in your life. If not you, you must have known people who begin a diet enthusiastically, then hit a plateau and give it all up in frustration and resume their unhealthy eating habits. Wondering what the DASH diet is all about? It's a one of a kind diet, specifically designed to reduce blood pressure levels in people. Hypertension, or high blood pressure, is one of the greatest silent killers of this century.

DASH stands for Dietary Approaches to Stop Hypertension. The DASH diet is rich in fruits, vegetables, whole grains, and low-fat dairy products. Its emphasis isn't on deprivation, but on adaptation. The DASH diet aims to change the way people look at food, to educate them about their bodies, and to teach them to make healthy, sustainable choices.

The DASH diet was created to change lives by changing lifestyles. Unlike more restrictive diets, the DASH diet was designed to be approachable, and to be readily incorporated into people's lives. For the most part, you do not need to shop at special grocery stores or go through agonizing transition periods; you just need to start adjusting your food patterns, one step at a time.

The basics of the DASH diet are simple: Eat more fruits, vegetables, whole grains, and lean protein, and eat less saturated fat, salt, and sweets. It's a common-sense approach to health that really works.

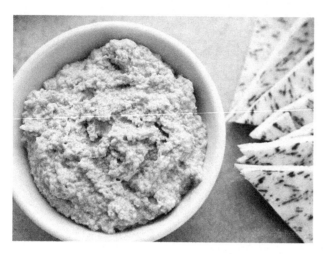

Why the DASH Diet Works

The DASH diet works because it's a lifestyle that can be sustained easily, not a traditional diet. The word "diet" conjures thoughts of temporary deprivation, but the DASH diet is the opposite. It aims at educating individuals on how they can undertake clean or proper eating, on a daily basis, so that they build healthy bodies. Rather than impose strict controls on food content, such as the total number of fat, DASH diet follows important rules of choosing clean foods. When individuals understand the implications of their daily dietary decision making, they're much more likely to choose wisely. Therefore, it is easy to adopt the DASH diet.

The ultimate goal of the DASH diet is to reduce the intake of harmful foods and to choose healthy substitutes instead. When you understand the damage that bad food does to your body, it makes you far less interested in eating it. And once you wean yourself from excess fat, cholesterol, sodium, and sugar, you will be amazed by how much better you feel! Bad food takes its toll in so many ways, not just silently with hypertension and heart disease, but also outwardly in your appearance, energy level, and enthusiasm for life. If you are feeling sluggish, consider what you last ate. Was it good for you? Or bad? Unless you are fueling your body with good food, it will fail you. The DASH diet isn't a strict dietary regimen, but rather a new way of seeing, appreciating, and consuming food.

Grains, vegetables, fruits, low-fat dairy products, seeds, nuts, and lean meat all form the base of the DASH diet. So, there are no strict restrictions, only amazing benefits. Besides giving you a way of turning to healthy eating habits, the DASH diet is primarily known for showing great results in lowering high blood pressure. This diet is rich in several minerals like calcium, zinc, iron, manganese, and potassium, and these nutrients primarily help to regulate the blood pressure. Also, the diet is low in saturated fat and cholesterol but provides a significant amount of protein, which can also help people suffering from high blood pressure.

Knowing what kind of foods make the foundation of this diet makes it clear that it can also be used to lose weight and excess fat. Following this kind of diet means losing about 500 calories a day. Combine that with exercise, and you will get slim fast. What supports this is also the fact that the DASH diet, rich in protein and fiber, keeps you satiated for longer periods and thus prevents overeating and gaining weight.

The DASH diet is one of the few diets that can help you meet your daily requirement for potassium, which, besides countering the effect of salt to raise blood pressure, also helps in preventing osteoporosis. This diet also provides sufficient amounts of vitamin B 12, calcium, and fiber, which are required for proper cell metabolism, building and maintaining strong bones, keeping blood sugar levels stable, and preventing obesity.

DASH Diet Benefits

Here are the advantages of going on a diet:

1. *Weight Loss-*

Obviously, the number one reason for embarking on any diet, weight loss not only gives you a pleasing appearance, it helps the body internally as well. Being overweight adds extra strain on your heart, liver, kidneys, joints and it also clogs your arteries. A balanced combination of diet and exercise will work wonders in giving you a whole new life. People put on weight simply because the number of calories they ingest is more than the number of calories they burn, plus a sedentary lifestyle. Instead of crash dieting, eat healthy and get regular exercise.

2. Lower Blood Pressure-

Losing between two and five percent of your extra weight will help lower your blood pressure and keep your diabetes under control. Extra weight equals more strain on the heart, and that means higher blood pressure.

3. Lower Triglycerides-

Triglycerides are important for your body, as they store any extra calories you consume. But constant storage of extra calories is what makes you fat. Higher levels of triglycerides are unhealthy for the heart and may cause coronary problems.

4. Improved cholesterol and a healthier heart-

A diet may help your good lipids, that is, your high-density lipoprotein (HDL), by boosting your metabolism and keeping your heart active. Plus, reducing your cholesterol levels, your bad lipid levels, increasing your metabolic rate and keeping your blood pressure under normal is vital for a healthy and properly functioning heart, cutting the risk of heart and coronary disease by a large margin.

5. Lower Glucose Levels-

Losing some weight can aid with the blood sugar levels in the body. This is great for the diabetics and those who wish to stay safe from the disease.

6. Improved Mood and Overall Fitness-

Not only does exercise and weight loss make you look good eventually, you will also begin to feel great and energetic throughout the day. Losing weight and keeping the body fit will result in an overall sense of well-being and energy, which no pill or juice can provide.

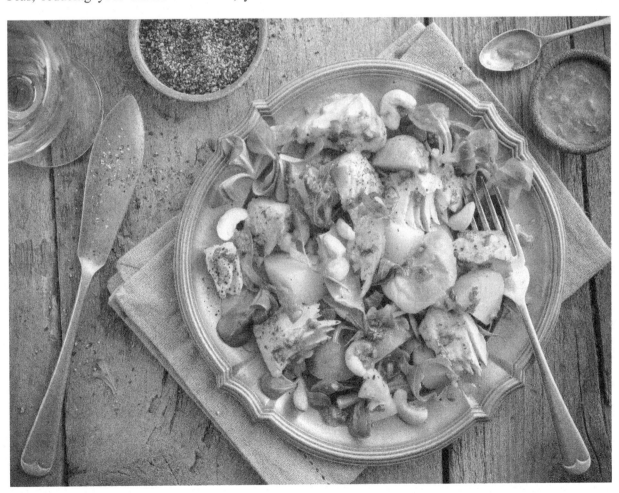

DASH Diet Health Plan

Dash diet for high blood pressure/hypertension

Your daily sodium intake from food should be between 1500 and 2300 milligrams per day. The latter is the highest level of sodium that is acceptable according to the National High Blood Pressure Education Program. This is also the amount that is recommended by the US Dietary Guidelines for Americans. 1500 Milligrams is the ideal amount of sodium per day according to the Institute of Medicine. This is the level that you should eventually strive for.

Blood pressure will gradually reduce as you reduce the amount of sodium you consume. DASH menus usually contain 2300 milligrams of sodium to help lower blood pressure gradually. On average, most men consume close to 4200 milligrams of sodium and women consume 3300 milligrams of sodium per day – which is significantly higher than the suggested levels.

The DASH diet consists of food that is low in sodium suitable for patients suffering from blood pressure. With DASH diet, you will experience multiple benefits that you can help you stabilize your blood pressure levels. When you follow a combination of a balanced eating plan and also work towards reducing the sodium content in food, you will be able to prevent the development of high blood pressure.

Dash diet for weight loss

Dash Diet indeed helps to trim your weight by various indirect means.

While the DASH diet does not focus on reducing calories, it fills up your diet with very nutrient dense foods as opposed to ones that are rich in calories, this helps to shed off a few pounds!

This diet is a great way to lose weight because it incorporates fresh, whole foods and reduces packaged, processed foods that are filled with empty calories. Not only will you lose weight, you'll also have a better chance of keeping it off.

DASH goes beyond the calorie counting and helps you establish sound eating habits that improve your chances for maintaining healthy weight.

Being on a diet full of veggies and fruits, you will consume lots of fiber, which is also believed to help in weight loss.

Apart from that, the diet also controls your appetite since cleaner and nutrition dense foods will keep you satisfied throughout the whole day. Lowering the food intake will further contribute to weight loss.

Steps Towards Transitioning to the DASH Diet

Changing your eating habits needs to be done gradually. Here are a few suggestions to help you make an easy transition to the DASH diet:

- Keep a journal and track your eating habits. What do you eat for breakfast, lunch, and dinner? How often do you eat in between meals, and what are you snacking on? From your journal, you can figure out where you need to make changes. For example, add a cup or two of vegetables and fruits to help reduce too many servings of meat. Limit your sodium and sugar by reading the nutrition facts labels on food packages.
- When shopping, choose "low-fat," "non-fat," "no sugar added," "no cholesterol," and other healthier versions of products. For grain servings, choose whole grains, such as whole wheat bread and whole grain cereals.
- If you love butter or margarine, decrease the amount you use by half and switch to no-cholesterol and low-sodium versions. You can use spices as a substitute for salt. Experiment with different herbs if you're not sure how they taste. Some examples of spices you can try are rosemary, basil, nutmeg, parsley, sage, and thyme.

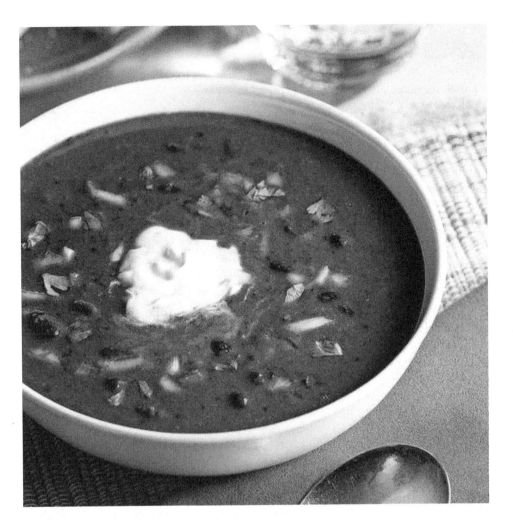

The do's and don'ts of Food

Good Foods for the DASH Diet

Whole grains

Whole grains must be carefully chosen for the DASH diet; they may include whole grain bread, pasta, cereals, and rice. Whole grains should constitute between 4 and 6 servings a day. An example of a serving of whole grain is ½ cup of rice or pasta. You should consider brown rice ahead of white rice because it contains more fiber. Likewise, consider whole grain bread instead of white bread because most white bread has refined components. Avoid bread made with butter and cream cheese.

Fruits and Vegetables

Fruits and vegetables should be consumed 4 - 5 times per day. Some of the best vegetables you can consider include tomatoes, sweet potatoes, broccoli, carrots, and green leafy vegetables such as spinach. ½ cup of cooked vegetables is a good example of a serving of vegetable. Frozen vegetables are much preferred to unfrozen because they increase your serving size. Make sure you choose low-sodium vegetables when you buy frozen products. ½ fresh or frozen or canned fruits, in natural juice, not surgery is also a good example of a serving.

For snacking, you can have a piece of fruit with a dollop of low-fat or non-fat yogurt. Make sure you consume the peels of fruits with edible peels such as pears, and apples because it contains fiber and other important essential nutrients. Juices of citrus fruits may interact with some medications, so be sure to confirm with your doctor before choosing such fruits.

Low or non-fat dairy

You may add low or non-fat dairy to your DASH diet if you are free from lactose intolerance. Milk, yogurts, and cheeses that are non-fat or low in fat, are healthy sources of calcium, protein and vitamin D. A cup of skim milk, a cup of non-fat yogurt, and 1 ounce of partly skim milk cheese, are also healthy examples of a serving of low fat dairy. Fat-free cheese products can be high in sodium, so you must go easy on them.

Lean meat, fish, and poultry

Meat recommended for the DASH diet must be lean. Meat provides crucial nutrients like iron and vitamin B. Lean meat should be consumed not more than 6 ounces a day. Make sure you trim away the fat from poultry meat and you can grill, boil, or roast your meat, try as much as possible to avoid frying. Mix heart-friendly fish species such as herring, salmon, or tuna, because they contain unsaturated fatty acid. Oily fishes in general contain Omega-3 fatty acids, known to reduce cholesterol.

Legumes, nuts, and seeds

Legumes, nuts, and seeds are rich in phytochemicals that reduce the risks of certain cardiovascular diseases and cancer. They also serve as good sources of essential minerals such as potassium, and magnesium, and provide substantial amounts of protein. The best nuts, seeds, and legumes you should consider for the DASH diet include peas, lentils, kidney beans, almonds, and sunflower seeds.

Serving sizes for legumes, nuts, and seeds should be small and they can be consumed a few days a week. A good example of a serving is 1/3 cup of groundnuts and ½ cup of cooked beans. Eat nuts in moderation, even though they contain omega-3 fatty acids that are good for the body. Tofu and tempeh are healthy alternatives to meat and contain protein and essential amino acids that the body needs.

You should consider 1 - 3 servings of fats a day; however, you must avoid trans-fats and saturated fats because they are the main triggers of numerous coronary heart diseases. Margarine and salad dressings are some of the easiest ways of consuming trans-fats; read food labels before purchasing.

Foods that Must be Avoided

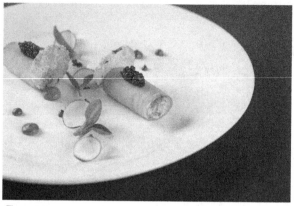

Sweets

Sweets should be consumed at less than 5 servings a week. When following the DASH diet, sweets are strictly prohibited, however, you don't have to banish them completely. If you must add some sweets to your diet, you could replace them with healthy substitutes, such as stevia and honey. You may occasionally add ½ cup of sorbet, 1 tablespoon of jelly or jam, or ½ a cup of lemonade.

If you can't avoid sweets completely, you may want to consider low or fat-free options such as sorbet, fruit ices, jelly beans, and low-fat cookies. You may also consider some artificial sweeteners such as aspartame, if you want to satisfy your sweet tooth; however, you need to ensure that you use them extremely sparingly. ½ - 2 tablespoons of artificial sweeteners may be used a week. Added sugar has no nutritional value and will add quite a few calories to your diet.

Carbonated soft drinks

Soft drinks, including soda, and other forms of sugary drinks must be avoided on the DASH diet because they are packed with empty sugary calories. The sugars in them are too easily absorbed into the blood stream and fat.

Alcohol and caffeinated drinks

Excessive consumption of alcohol can lead to a sharp increase in blood pressure. For this reason, alcohol should be avoided, or at most reduce consumption. (As noted in previous chapter.) If caffeinated drinks, such as coffee cause decline or increase in your blood pressure, you should avoid caffeine as well.

Processed foods

Processed foods, especially carb-loaded foods, should be avoided. These include white flour, as well as baked confectioneries that are heavily loaded with calories. Substitute all processed foods with whole and unprocessed ones.

Creating a Meal Plan

Starting a DASH diet requires that you set a goal, however your goal must be realistic. Keep in mind the DASH diet is not a quick weight loss program, but a permanent lifestyle program that should be sustained over a period of time. Once you set a goal, you must stick with it and devise a method to achieve your goal.

#1: Aim at losing 1 - 5 pounds every week – If you are looking at losing more than 20 pounds a month, then this may not be the plan for you. Researchers have shown that people who follow the DASH diet from the start are able to lose between 1 - 5 pounds on a weekly basis, depending on how their metabolism metabolizes, and how well they substitute unhealthy food components with healthy ones.

#2: Before you start a DASH diet, make sure you clean out your refrigerator and kitchen cabinets – remove unhealthy foods and start replacing them with healthy and organic food. Make sure you shop for foods that will last for weeks, if not months, and prepare as many of them as you can.

#3: If you are a busy, working class individual, it will be ideal to prepare your meals in bulk, this will help you save time in the long run, and make your DASH diet plan a lot easier to maintain.

#4: If you find it difficult to eliminate all unhealthy foods you are addicted to, at the same time, you can set out a pre-DASH period where you eliminate each unhealthy food one at a time, until you have healthy foods recommended through the DASH diet. Take your time to check for sugar alternatives, and healthier alternatives that will contribute fewer calories to your diet.

#5: Take affirmative action on how you are going to achieve your weight loss strategy. Remember, the DASH diet does not encourage you to put your body in fast mode, because fasting cannot cause weight loss.

Utensils and Cookware

- ✓ **_Choose the right cookware:_** Make sure that you have the appropriate cookware and gadgets in place. This will help you prepare your DASH diet recipes with ease. Some of the cookware that need to find a place in your kitchen are as follows:
- ✓ **_- Nonstick cookware:_** When you use nonstick cookware, you will end up using less oil or butter while cooking your meat or vegetables. You can also make use of non-stick spray that will replace your oils and butters. But make sure you make use of the best and quality products as some might be of poor quality. Buy the best brands and your investment will be fruitful.
- ✓ **_- Pressure cooker:_** it is a good idea for you to buy yourself a pressure cooker. A pressure cooker will help you cook your meals with ease. You don't have to put in too much effort towards it and only have to wait on it to blow a few whistles. The steam will cook the ingredients and you can eat your meal.
- ✓ **_- Slow cooker:_** better known as a crock pot, a slow cooker will help you cook a meal at a slow speed which will help in preserving the nutrients in the meal. You can buy a crock-pot online and use it to cook your food. The slow cooker you buy will come with the instructions to operate it that you can see and use.
- ✓ **_- Instant Pot:_** Helps you to prepare meals when in a rush.
- ✓ **_- Garlic press or spice mill:_** Most of us tend to add salt at the table, to add more flavors to our food. These items will help you add more flavors to your food. Hence, this will discourage you from adding salt to your food at the table.
- ✓ **_- Vegetable steamer insert:_** When you have a vegetable steamer insert, which you can fit into the bottom of a saucepan, you will find it easier to prepare steamed vegetables, without adding oil or butter to the pan.
- ✓ **_- Sprouter:_** A Sprouter is a device that you can use to sprout the lentils and beans. It will help you sprout them and you can easily add it to your salads.

Chapter 2 Breakfast Recipes

Sweet Potatoes with Coconut Flakes

Prep time: 15 mins | Servings: 2

Ingredients:
- 16 oz. sweet potatoes
- 1 tbsp. maple syrup
- ¼ c. fat-free coconut Greek yogurt
- 1/8 c. unsweetened toasted coconut flakes
- 1 chopped apple

Directions:
1. Preheat oven to 400 °F.
2. Place your potatoes on a baking sheet. Bake them for 45 - 60 minutes or until soft.
3. Use a sharp knife to mark "X" on the potatoes and fluff pulp with a fork.
4. Top with coconut flakes, chopped apple, Greek yogurt, and maple syrup.
5. Serve immediately.

Nutritional Information:
Calories: 321, Fat: 3 g, Carbs: 70 g, Protein: 7 g, Sugars: 0.1 g, Sodium: 599 mg

Flaxseed & Banana Smoothie

Prep time: 5 mins | Servings: 1

Ingredients:
- 1 frozen banana
- ½ c. almond milk
- Vanilla extract.
- 2 tbsps. Flax seed
- 1 tsp. maple syrup
- 1 tbsp. almond butter

Directions:
1. Add all your ingredients to a food processor or blender and run until smooth.
2. Pour the mixture into a glass and enjoy.

Nutritional Information:
Calories: 376, Fat:19.4 g, Carbs:48.3 g, Protein:9.2 g, Sugars:20.6 g, Sodium:64.9 mg

Fruity Tofu Smoothie

Prep time: 5 mins | Servings: 2

Ingredients:
- 1 c. ice cold water
- 1 c. packed spinach
- ¼ c. frozen mango chunks
- ½ c. frozen pineapple chunks
- 1 tbsp. chia seeds
- 1 container silken tofu
- 1 frozen medium banana

Directions:
1. In a powerful blender, add all ingredients and puree until smooth and creamy.
2. Evenly divide into two glasses, serve and enjoy.

Nutritional Information:
Calories: 175, Fat:3.7 g, Carbs:33.3 g, Protein:6.0 g, Sugars:16.3 g, Sodium:24.1 mg

French Toast with Applesauce

Prep time: 5 mins | Servings: 6

Ingredients:
- ¼ c. unsweetened applesauce
- ½ c. skim milk
- 2 packets Stevia
- 2 eggs
- 6 slices whole wheat bread
- 1 tsp. ground cinnamon

Directions:
1. Mix well applesauce, sugar, cinnamon, milk and eggs in a mixing bowl.
2. One slice at a time, soak the bread into applesauce mixture until wet.
3. On medium fire, heat a large nonstick skillet.
4. Add soaked bread on one side and another on the other side. Cook in a single layer in batches for 2-3 minutes per side on medium low fire or until lightly browned.
5. Serve and enjoy.

Nutritional Information:
Calories: 122.6, Fat:2.6 g, Carbs:18.3 g, Protein:6.5 g, Sugars:14.8 g, Sodium231: mg

Banana-Peanut Butter 'n Greens Smoothie

Prep time: 5 mins | Servings: 1

Ingredients:
- 1 c. chopped and packed Romaine lettuce
- 1 frozen medium banana
- 1 tbsp. all-natural peanut butter
- 1 c. cold almond milk

Directions:
1. In a heavy-duty blender, add all ingredients.
2. Puree until smooth and creamy.
3. Serve and enjoy.

Nutritional Information:
Calories: 349.3, Fat:9.7 g, Carbs:57.4 g, Protein:8.1 g, Sugars:4.3 g, Sodium:151 mg

Baking Powder Biscuits

Prep time: 5 mins | Servings: 1

Ingredients:
- 1 egg white
- 1 c. white whole-wheat flour
- 4 tbsps. Non-hydrogenated vegetable shortening
- 1 tbsp. sugar
- 2/3 c. low-fat milk
- 1 c. unbleached all-purpose flour
- 4 tsps. Sodium-free baking powder

Directions:
1. Preheat oven to 450°F. Take out a baking sheet and set aside.
2. Place the flour, sugar, and baking powder into a mixing bowl and whisk well to combine.
3. Cut the shortening into the mixture using your fingers, and work until it resembles coarse crumbs. Add the egg white and milk and stir to combine.
4. Turn the dough out onto a lightly floured surface and knead 1 minute. Roll dough to ¾ inch thickness and cut into 12 rounds.
5. Place rounds on the baking sheet. Place baking sheet on middle rack in oven and bake 10 minutes.
6. Remove baking sheet and place biscuits on a wire rack to cool.

Nutritional Information:
Calories: 118, Fat:4 g, Carbs:16 g, Protein:3 g, Sugars:0.2 g, Sodium: 294mg

Oatmeal Banana Pancakes with Walnuts

Prep time: 15 mins | Servings: 8 pancakes

Ingredients:
- 1 finely diced firm banana
- 1 c. whole wheat pancake mix
- 1/8 c. chopped walnuts
- ¼ c. old-fashioned oats

Directions:
1. Make the pancake mix according to the directions on the package.
2. Add walnuts, oats, and chopped banana.
3. Coat a griddle with cooking spray. Add about ¼ cup of the pancake batter onto the griddle when hot.
4. Turn pancake over when bubbles form on top. Cook until golden brown.
5. Serve immediately.

Nutritional Information:
Calories: 155, Fat:4 g, Carbs:28 g, Protein:7 g, Sugars:2.2 g, Sodium:320 mg

Creamy Oats, Greens & Blueberry Smoothie

Prep time: 4 mins | Servings: 1

Ingredients:
- 1 c. cold fat-free milk
- 1 c. salad greens
- ½ c. fresh frozen blueberries
- ½ c. frozen cooked oatmeal
- 1 tbsp. sunflower seeds

Directions:
1. In a powerful blender, blend all ingredients until smooth and creamy.
2. Serve and enjoy.

Nutritional Information:
Calories: 280, Fat:6.8 g, Carbs:44.0 g, Protein:14.0 g, Sugars:32 g, Sodium:242 mg

Banana & Cinnamon Oatmeal

Prep time: 5 mins | Servings: 6

Ingredients:
- 2 c. quick-cooking oats
- 4 c. fat-free milk
- 1 tsp. ground cinnamon
- 2 chopped large ripe banana
- 4 tsps. Brown sugar
- Extra ground cinnamon

Directions:
1. Place milk in a skillet and bring to boil. Add oats and cook over medium heat until thickened, for two to four minutes. Stir intermittently.
2. Add cinnamon, brown sugar and banana and stir to combine.
3. If you want, serve with the extra cinnamon and milk.
4. Enjoy!

Nutritional Information:
Calories: 215, Fat:2 g, Carbs:42 g, Protein:10 g, Sugars:1 g, Sodium:98 mg

Bagels Made Healthy

Prep time: 5 mins | Servings: 8

Ingredients:
- 1 ½ c. warm water
- 1 ¼ c. bread flour
- 2 tbsps. Honey
- 2 c. whole wheat flour
- 2 tsps. Yeast
- 1 ½ tbsps. Olive oil
- 1 tbsp. vinegar

Directions:
1. In a bread machine, mix all ingredients, and then process on dough cycle.

2. Once done, create 8 pieces shaped like a flattened ball.
3. Make a hole in the center of each ball using your thumb then create a donut shape.
4. In a greased baking sheet, place donut-shaped dough then cover and let it rise about ½ hour.
5. Prepare about 2 inches of water to boil in a large pan.
6. In a boiling water, drop one at a time the bagels and boil for 1 minute, then turn them once.
7. Remove them and return to baking sheet and bake at 350oF for about 20 to 25 minutes until golden brown.

Nutritional Information:
Calories: 228.1, Fat:3.7 g, Carbs:41.8 g, Protein:6.9 g, Sugars:0 g, Sodium:499 mg

Cereal with Cranberry-Orange Twist

Prep time: 5 mins | Servings: 1

Ingredients:
- ½ c. water
- ½ c. orange juice
- 1/3 c. oat bran
- ¼ c. dried cranberries
- Sugar
- Milk

Directions:
1. In a bowl, combine all ingredients.
2. For about 2 minutes, microwave the bowl then serve with sugar and milk.
3. Enjoy!

Nutritional Information:
Calories: 220.4, Fat:2.4 g, Carbs:43.5 g, Protein:6.2 g, Sugars:8 g, Sodium:110 mg

No Cook Overnight Oats

Prep time: 5 mins | Servings: 1

Ingredients:
- 1 ½ c. low fat milk
- 5 whole almond pieces
- 1 tsp. chia seeds
- 2 tbsps. Oats
- 1 tsp. sunflower seeds
- 1 tbsp. Craisins

Directions:
1. In a jar or mason bottle with cap, mix all ingredients.
2. Refrigerate overnight.
3. Enjoy for breakfast. Will keep in the fridge for up to 3 days.

Nutritional Information:
Calories: 271, Fat:9.8 g, Carbs:35.4 g, Protein:16.7 g, Sugars:9 g, Sodium:97 mg

Avocado Cup with Egg

Prep time: 5 mins | Servings: 4

Ingredients:
- 4 tsps. parmesan cheese
- 1 chopped stalk scallion
- 4 dashes pepper
- 4 dashes paprika
- 2 ripe avocados
- 4 medium eggs

Directions:
1. Preheat oven to 375 °F.
2. Slice avocadoes in half and discard seed.
3. Slice the rounded portions of the avocado, to make it level and sit well on a baking sheet.
4. Place avocadoes on baking sheet and crack one egg in each hole of the avocado.
5. Season each egg evenly with pepper, and paprika.
6. Pop in the oven and bake for 25 minutes or until eggs are cooked to your liking.
7. Serve with a sprinkle of parmesan.

Nutritional Information:
Calories: 206, Fat:15.4 g, Carbs:11.3 g, Protein:8.5 g, Sugars:0.4 g, Sodium:380 mg

Mediterranean Toast

Prep time: 10 mins | Servings: 2

Ingredients:
- 1 ½ tsp. reduced-fat crumbled feta
- 3 sliced Greek olives
- ¼ mashed avocado
- 1 slice good whole wheat bread
- 1 tbsp. roasted red pepper hummus
- 3 sliced cherry tomatoes
- 1 sliced hardboiled egg

Directions:
1. First, toast the bread and top it with ¼ mashed avocado and 1 tablespoon hummus.
2. Add the cherry tomatoes, olives, hardboiled egg, and feta.
3. To taste, season with salt and pepper.

Nutritional Information:
Calories: 333.7, Fat:17 g, Carbs:33.3 g, Protein:16.3 g, Sugars:1 g, Sodium:700 mg

Instant Banana Oatmeal

Prep time: 1 min | Servings: 1

Ingredients:
- 1 mashed ripe banana
- ½ c. water
- ½ c. quick oats

Directions:
1. Measure the oats and water into a microwave-safe bowl and stir to combine.
2. Place bowl in microwave and heat on high for 2 minutes.
3. Remove bowl from microwave and stir in the mashed banana and enjoy.

Nutritional Information:
Calories: 243, Fat:3 g, Carbs:50 g, Protein:6 g, Sugars:20 g, Sodium:30 mg

Almond Butter-Banana Smoothie

Prep time: 5 mins | Servings: 1

Ingredients:
- 1 tbsp. almond butter
- ½ c. ice cubes
- ½ c. packed spinach
- 1 peeled and frozen medium banana
- 1 c. fat-free milk

Directions:
1. In a powerful blender, blend all ingredients until smooth and creamy.
2. Serve and enjoy.

Nutritional Information:
Calories: 293, Fat:9.8 g, Carbs:42.5 g, Protein:13.5 g, Sugars:12 g, Sodium:111 mg

Brown Sugar Cinnamon Oatmeal

Prep time: 1 min | Servings: 4

Ingredients:
- ½ tsp. ground cinnamon
- 1 ½ tsps. pure vanilla extract
- ¼ c. light brown sugar
- 2 c. low-fat milk
- 1 1/3 c. quick oats

Directions:
1. Measure the milk and vanilla into a medium saucepan and bring to a boil over medium-high heat.
2. Once boiling, reduce heat to medium. Stir in oats, brown sugar, and cinnamon, and cook, stirring, 2–3 minutes.
3. Serve immediately, sprinkled with additional cinnamon if desired.

Nutritional Information:
Calories: 208, Fat:3 g, Carbs:38 g, Protein:8 g, Sugars:15 g, Sodium:105 mg

Buckwheat Pancakes with Vanilla Almond Milk

Prep time: 10 mins | Servings: 1

Ingredients:
- ½ c. unsweetened vanilla almond milk
- 2-4 packets natural sweetener
- 1/8 tsp. salt
- ½ cup buckwheat flour
- ½ tsp. double-acting baking powder

Directions:
1. Prepare a nonstick pancake griddle and spray with the cooking spray, place over medium heat.
2. Whisk together the buckwheat flour, salt, baking powder, and stevia in a small bowl and stir in the almond milk after.
3. Onto the pan, scoop a large spoonful of batter, cook until bubbles no longer pop on the surface and the entire surface looks dry and (2-4 minutes). Flip and cook for another 2-4 minutes. Repeat with all the remaining batter.

Nutritional Information:
Calories: 240, Fat:4.5 g, Carbs:2 g, Protein:11 g, Sugars:17 g, Sodium:67 mg

Tomato Bruschetta with Basil

Prep time: 10 mins | Servings: 8

Ingredients:
- ½ c. chopped basil
- 2 minced garlic cloves
- 1 tbsp. balsamic vinegar
- 2 tbsps. Olive oil
- ½ tsp. cracked black pepper
- 1 sliced whole wheat baguette
- 8 diced ripe Roma tomatoes
- 1 tsp. sea salt

Directions:
1. First, preheat the oven to 375 F.
2. In a bowl, dice the tomatoes, mix in balsamic vinegar, chopped basil, garlic, salt, pepper, and olive oil, set aside.
3. Slice the baguette into 16-18 slices and for about 10 minutes, place on a baking pan to bake.
4. Serve with warm bread slices and enjoy.
5. For leftovers, store in an airtight container and put in the fridge. Try putting them over grilled chicken, it is amazing!

Nutritional Information:
Calories: 57, Fat:2.5 g, Carbs:7.9 g, Protein:1.4 g, Sugars:0.2 g, Sodium:261 mg

Sweet Corn Muffins

Prep time: 5 mins | Servings: 1

Ingredients:
- 1 tbsp. sodium-free baking powder
- ¾ c. nondairy milk
- 1 tsp. pure vanilla extract
- ½ c. sugar
- 1 c. white whole-wheat flour
- 1 c. cornmeal
- ½ c. canola oil

Directions:
1. Preheat the oven to 400°F. Line a 12-muffin tin with paper liners and set aside.
2. Place the cornmeal, flour, sugar, and baking powder into a mixing bowl and whisk well to combine.
3. Add the nondairy milk, oil, and vanilla and stir just until combined.
4. Divide the batter evenly between the muffin cups. Place muffin tin on middle rack in oven and bake for 15 minutes.
5. Remove from oven and place on a wire rack to cool.

Nutritional Information:
Calories: 203, Fat:9 g, Carbs:26 g, Protein:3 g, Sugars:9.5 g, Sodium:255 mg

Scrambled Eggs with Mushrooms and Spinach

Prep time: 5 mins | Servings: 1

Ingredients:
- 2 egg whites
- 1 slice whole wheat toast
- ½ c. sliced fresh mushrooms
- 2 tbsps. Shredded fat free American cheese
- Pepper
- 1 tsp. olive oil
- 1 c. chopped fresh spinach
- 1 whole egg

Directions:
1. On medium high fire, place a nonstick fry pan and add oil. Swirl oil to cover pan and heat for a minute.
2. Add spinach and mushrooms. Sauté until spinach is wilted, around 2-3 minutes.
3. Meanwhile, in a bowl whisk well egg, egg whites, and cheese. Season with pepper.
4. Pour egg mixture into pan and scramble until eggs are cooked through, around 3-4 minutes.
5. Serve and enjoy with a piece of whole wheat toast.

Nutritional Information:
Calories: 290.6, Fat:11.8 g, Carbs:21.8 g, Protein:24.3 g, Sugars:1.4 g, Sodium:1000 mg

Chia and Oat Breakfast Bran

Prep time: overnight | Servings: 2

Ingredients:
- 85 g chopped roasted almonds
- 340 g coconut milk
- 30 g cane sugar
- 2½ g orange zest
- 30 g flax seed mix
- 170 g rolled oats
- 340 g blueberries
- 30 g chia seeds
- 2½ g cinnamon

Directions:
1. Add all your wet ingredients together and mix the sugar and milk in with the orange zest.
2. Stir in the cinnamon and mix well. Once you are sure the sugar isn't lumpy add in the rolled oats, flax seeds, and chia and then let it sit for a minute.
3. Grab two bowls or mason jars and pour the mixture in. Top with the roasted almonds, and store in the fridge.
4. Pull it out in the morning and dig in!

Nutritional Information:
Calories: 353, Fat:8 g, Carbs:55 g, Protein:15 g, Sugars:9.9 g, Sodium:96 mg

Faux Breakfast Hash Brown Cups

Prep time: 15 mins | Servings: 8

Ingredients:
- 40 g diced onion
- 8 large eggs
- 7 ½ g garlic powder
- 2 ½ g pepper
- 170 g shredded low-fat cheese
- 170 g grated sweet potato
- 2 ½ g salt

Directions:
1. Preheat oven to 400 °F and prepare a muffin tin with liners.
2. Place grated sweet potatoes, onions, garlic, and spices into a bowl and mix well, before placing one spoonful in each cup. Add one large egg upon each cup and proceed to bake for 15 minutes until eggs are cooked.
3. Serve fresh or store.

Nutritional Information:
Calories: 143, Fat:9.1 g, Carbs:6 g, Protein:9 g, Sugars:0 g, Sodium:290 mg

Maple Mocha Frappe

Prep time: 2 mins | Servings: 2

Ingredients:
- 1 tbsp. unsweetened cocoa powder
- ½ c. low-fat milk
- 2 tbsps. Pure maple syrup
- ½ c. brewed coffee
- 1 small ripe banana
- 1 c. low-fat vanilla yogurt

Directions:
1. Place the banana in a blender or food processor and purée.
2. Add the remaining ingredients and pulse until smooth and creamy.
3. Serve immediately.

Nutritional Information:
Calories: 206, Fat:2 g, Carbs:38 g, Protein:6 g, Sugars:17 g, Sodium:65 mg

Breakfast Oatmeal in Slow Cooker

Prep time: 10 mins | Servings: 8

Ingredients:
- 4 c. almond milk
- 2 packets stevia
- 2 c. steel-cut oats
- 1/3 c. chopped dried apricots
- 4 c. water
- 1/3 c. dried cherries
- 1 tsp. cinnamon
- 1/3 c. raisins

Directions:
1. In slow cooker, mix well all ingredients.
2. Cover and set to low.
3. Cook for 8 hours.
4. You can set this the night before so that by morning you have breakfast ready.

Nutritional Information:
Calories: 158.5, Fat:2.9 g, Carbs:28.3 g, Protein:4.8 g, Sugars:11 g, Sodium:135 mg

Apple Cinnamon Overnight Oats

Prep time: 15 mins | Servings: 2

Ingredients:
- 1 diced apple
- 2 tbsps. Chia seeds
- ½ tbsp. ground cinnamon
- ½ tsp. pure vanilla extract
- 1¼ c. nonfat milk
- Kosher salt
- 1 c. old-fashioned rolled oats
- 2 tsps. Honey

Directions:
1. Divide the oats, chia seeds or ground flaxseed, milk, cinnamon, honey or maple syrup, vanilla extract, and salt into two Mason jars. Place the lids tightly on top and shake until thoroughly combined.
2. Remove the lids and add half of the diced apple to each jar. Sprinkle with additional cinnamon, if desired. Place the lids tightly back on the jars and refrigerate for at least 4 hours or overnight.
3. You can store the overnight oats in single-serve containers in the refrigerator for up to 3 days.

Nutritional Information:
Calories: 339, Fat:8 g, Carbs:60 g, Protein:13 g, Sugars:15 g, Sodium:161 mg.

Hot Honey Porridge

Prep time: 5 mins | Servings: 4

Ingredients:
- ¼ c. honey
- ½ c. rolled oats
- 3 c. boiling water
- ¾ c. bulgur wheat

Directions:
1. Place the bulgur wheat and rolled oats into a saucepan. Add the boiling water and stir to combine.
2. Place pan over high heat and bring to a boil. Once boiling, reduce heat to low, then cover and simmer for 10 minutes, stirring occasionally.
3. Remove from heat, stir in honey, and serve immediately.

Nutritional Information:
Calories: 172, Fat:1 g, Carbs:40 g, Protein:4 g, Sugars:5 g, Sodium:20 mg

French Toast with Cinnamon Vanilla

Prep time: 5 mins | Servings: 4

Ingredients:
- ½ tsp. cinnamon
- 3 large eggs
- 1 tsp. vanilla
- 8 whole-wheat slices bread
- 2 tbsps. Low-fat milk

Directions:
1. First, preheat a griddle to 350°F.
2. Combine the vanilla, eggs, milk, and cinnamon in a small bowl and whisk until smooth.
3. Pour into a plate or flat-bottomed dish.
4. Into the egg mixture, dip the bread, flip to coat both sides and put on the hot griddle.
5. Cook for about 2 minutes or until the bottom is lightly browned, then flip and cook the other side as well.

Nutritional Information:
Calories: 281.0, Fat:10.8 g, Carbs:37.2 g, Protein:14.5 g, Sugars:10 g, Sodium:390 mg.

Breakfast Grains and Fruits

Prep time: 10 mins | Servings: 6

Ingredients:
- 1 c. raisins
- ¾ c. quick cooking brown rice
- 1 granny smith apple
- 1 orange
- 8 oz. low fat vanilla yogurt
- 3 c. water
- ¾ c. bulgur
- 1 red delicious apple

Directions:
1. On high fire, place a large pot and bring water to a boil.
2. Add bulgur and rice. Lower fire to a simmer and cook for ten minutes while covered.
3. Turn off fire, set aside for 2 minutes while covered.
4. In baking sheet, transfer and evenly spread grains to cool.
5. Meanwhile, peel oranges and cut into sections. Chop and core apples.
6. Once grains are cool, transfer to a large serving bowl along with fruits.
7. Add yogurt and mix well to coat.
8. Serve and enjoy.

Nutritional Information:
Calories: 121, Fat:1 g, Carbs:24.2 g, Protein:3.8 g, Sugars:4.2 g, Sodium:500 mg

Eggs with Cheese

Prep time: 5 mins | Servings: 1

Ingredients:
- ¼ c. chopped tomato
- 1 egg white
- 1 chopped green onion
- 2 tbsps. Fat-free milk
- 1 slice whole wheat bread
- 1 egg
- ½ oz. reduced fat grated cheddar cheese

Directions:
1. Mix the egg and egg whites in a bowl and add the milk.
2. Scramble the mixture in a non-stick frying pan until the eggs cook.
3. Meanwhile, toast the bread.
4. Spoon the scrambled egg mixture onto the toasted bread and top with the cheese until it melts.
5. Add the onion and the tomato.

Nutritional Information:
Calories: 251, Fat:11.0 g, Carbs:22.3 g, Protein:16.9 g, Sugars:1.8 g, Sodium:451 mg

Hearty Orange Peach Smoothie

Prep time: 5 mins | Servings: 2

Ingredients:
- 2 c. chopped peaches
- 2 tbsps. Unsweetened yogurt
- Juice of 2 oranges

Directions:
1. Start by removing the seeds and peel from the peaches. Chop and leave some chunks of peach for topping.
2. Place the chopped peach, orange juice and yogurt in a blender and run until smooth.
3. You may add some water to thin the smoothie if you want.
4. Pour into glass cups and enjoy!

Nutritional Information:
Calories: 170, Fat:4.5 g, Carbs:28 g, Protein:7 g, Sugars:23 g, Sodium:101 mg

Cheddar & Kale Frittata

Prep time: 10 mins | Servings: 6

Ingredients:
- 1/3 c. sliced scallions
- ¼ tsp. pepper
- 1 diced red pepper
- ¾ c. non-fat milk
- 1 c. shredded sharp low-fat cheddar cheese
- 1 tsp. olive oil
- 5 oz. baby kale and spinach
- 12 eggs

Directions:
1. Preheat oven to 375 °F.
2. With olive oil, grease a glass casserole dish.
3. In a bowl, whisk well all ingredients except for cheese.
4. Pour egg mixture in prepared dish and bake for 35 minutes.
5. Remove from oven and sprinkle cheese on top and broil for 5 minutes.
6. Remove from oven and let it sit for 10 minutes.
7. Cut up and enjoy.

Nutritional Information:
Calories: 198, Fat:11.0 g, Carbs:5.7 g, Protein:18.7 g, Sugars:1 g, Sodium:209 mg

Spinach Mushroom Omelette

Prep time: 5 mins | Servings: 2

Ingredients:
- 2 tbsps. Olive oil
- 2 whole eggs
- 3 c. spinach, fresh
- Cooking spray
- 10 sliced baby Bella mushrooms
- 8 tbsps. Sliced red onion
- 4 egg whites
- 2 oz. goat cheese

Directions:
1. Place a skillet over medium-high heat and add olive.
2. Add the sliced red onions to the pan and stir until translucent. Then, add your mushrooms to the pan and keep stirring until they are slightly brown.
3. Add spinach and stir until they wilted. Season with a tiny bit of pepper and salt. Remove from heat.
4. Spray a small pan with cooking spray and Place over medium heat.
5. Break 2 whole eggs in a small bowl. Add 4 egg whites and whisk to combine.
6. Pour the whisked eggs into the small skillet and allow the mixture to sit for a minute.
7. Use a spatula to gently work your way around the skillet's edges. Raise the skillet and tip it down and around in a circular style to allow the runny eggs to reach the center and cook around the edges of the skillet.
8. Add crumbled goat cheese to a side of the omelet top with your mushroom mixture.
9. Then, gently fold the other side of the omelet over the mushroom side with the spatula.
10. Allowing cooking for thirty seconds. Then, transfer the omelet to a plate.

Nutritional Information:
Calories: 412, Fat:29 g, Carbs:18 g, Protein:25 g, Sugars:7 g, Sodium:1000 mg

Spinach 'n Tomato Egg Scramble

Prep time: 5 mins | Servings: 1

Ingredients:
- 1 tsp. olive oil
- 1 tsp. chopped fresh basil
- 1 medium chopped tomato
- ¼ c. Swiss cheese
- 2 eggs
- ½ tsp. cayenne pepper
- ½ c. chopped packed spinach

Directions:
1. In a small bowl, whisk well eggs, basil, pepper, and Swiss cheese.
2. Place a medium fry pan on medium fire and heat oil.
3. Stir in tomato and sauté for 3 minutes. Stir in spinach and cook for 2 minutes or until starting to wilt.
4. Pour in beaten eggs and scramble for 2 to 3 minutes or to desired doneness.
5. Enjoy.

Nutritional Information:
Calories: 230, Fat:14.3 g, Carbs:8.4 g, Protein:17.9 g, Sugars:1 g, Sodium:247 mg.

Mango and Coconut Oatmeal

Prep time: 10 mins | Servings: 1

Ingredients:
- ½ c. coconut milk
- Kosher salt
- 1 c. old-fashioned rolled oats
- 1/3 c. fresh chopped mango
- 2 tbsps. Unsweetened coconut flakes

Directions:

1. Bring the milk to a boil in a medium saucepan over high heat. Stir in the oats and salt and reduce the heat to low. Simmer for about 5 minutes, until the oats are creamy and tender.
2. In the meantime, toast coconut flakes for about 2 - 3 minutes until golden in a small dry skillet over low heat.
3. Once done, top the oatmeal with mango and coconut flakes, serve, and enjoy.

Nutritional Information:
Calories: 428, Fat:18 g, Carbs:60 g, Protein:10 g, Sugars:26 g, Sodium:122 mg.

Hearty Green Smoothie

Prep time: 5 mins | Servings: 4

Ingredients:
- 4 c. frozen mango
- 2 tsps. Ginger root
- 4 tbsps. Fresh lemon juice
- 2 c. fresh baby spinach, fresh
- 20 fresh peppermint leaves
- 2 c. English cucumber
- 1 jalapeno pepper
- 1½ c. water or unsweetened iced green tea

Directions:
1. Cube your frozen mango and add into a blender.
2. Chop cucumber and add into the blender.
3. Add the remaining ingredients, cover, and blend.
4. Enjoy!

Nutritional Information:
Calories: 142, Fat:0 g, Carbs:35 g, Protein:1 g, Sugars:16 g, Sodium:75 mg

Quick Turmeric Oatmeal

Prep time: 5 mins | Servings: 2

Ingredients:
- 2 c. water
- 1 tsp. turmeric powder
- Mint leaves
- 1 c. whole rolled oats
- 2 splashes oat milk

Directions:
1. Place your rolled oats in a bowl.
2. Add turmeric powder, milk and water and stir to mix.
3. Add toppings and cover.
4. Place in the fridge overnight.
5. Enjoy a glowing breakfast bowl in the morning.

Nutritional Information:
Calories: 154.6, Fat:3.1 g, Carbs:29.2 g, Protein:5.1 g, Sugars:2 g, Sodium:5.2 mg

Berry Bowl

Prep time: 5 mins | Servings: 2

Ingredients:
- ¼ c. fresh blueberries
- 1/3 c. unsweetened almond milk
- 2 tbsps. Unsweetened whey protein powder
- 2 c. frozen blueberries
- ¼ c. fat-free plain Greek yogurt

Directions:
1. In a blender, add blueberries and pulse for about 1 minute.
2. Add almond milk, yogurt, and protein powder and pulse until desired consistency.
3. Transfer the mixture into 2 serving bowls, dividing evenly.
4. Serve topped with fresh blueberries.

Nutritional Information:
Calories: 160, Fat:1.8 g, Carbs:23.5 g, Protein:15.3 g, Sugars:36 g, Sodium:60 mg

Delicious Flaxseed Banana Porridge

Prep time: 5 mins | Servings: 2

Ingredients:

For porridge:
- ½ c. ground flaxseeds
- 2¼ c. non-dairy milk
- ¼ tsp. sea salt
- ½ tsp. ground cinnamon
- 2 mashed banana

For topping:
- Pure maple syrup
- Fresh blueberries
- Chopped raw walnuts

Directions:

1. Place all the porridge ingredients in a medium skillet and mix to combine.
2. Place the pan over medium heat and stir continuously until the mixture reaches a low boil and becomes thick, about five minutes.
3. Remove from heat and place the porridge in a serving bowl.
4. Top your porridge with a little handful of walnuts and blueberries and enjoy warm!

Nutritional Information:
Calories: 155.6, Fat:9.1 g, Carbs:13.3 g, Protein:9.2 g, Sugars:2.4 g, Sodium:115 mg

Greens and Ginger Smoothie

Prep time: 5 mins | Servings: 4

Ingredients:
- 4 whole chopped stalks celery
- 40 g raw ginger
- 2 unpeeled and sliced medium cucumbers
- Crushed ice
- 340 g mixed kale
- 1 whole lemon
- 3 medium granny smith apples
- 680 g orange juice

Directions:
1. Add ginger to jazz things up.
2. Add the greens to the blender; the kale, the sliced cucumbers, the celery and the chopped apples.
3. Let them blend for about a minute while you peel a lemon, or just juice it if you want.
4. Add the lemon peel or juice and add in the chopped ginger.
5. Blend and top with ice and you are ready!

Nutritional Information:
Calories: 121, Fat:0.7 g, Carbs:26.64 g, Protein:4 g, Sugars:30 g, Sodium:50 mg

Peanut Butter with Chia Seeds Overnight Oats

Prep time: 5 mins | Servings: 2

Ingredients:
- 1 c. unsweetened plain almond milk
- 2 tbsps. Maple syrup
- Sliced banana
- 4 tbsps. Almond butter
- 1 c. gluten-free rolled oats
- 1½ tbsps. Chia seeds

Directions:
1. Add maple syrup, almond/peanut butter, chia seeds, and almond milk to a bowl. Stir to with a spoon until mixed.
2. Stir in the oats and press down with a spoon to make sure all the oats are immersed in the milk.
3. Cover the mixture tightly and place in the refrigerator overnight or for a minimum of six hours.
4. Enjoy as it is in the morning or top with sliced banana before eating.
5. You can refrigerate left over for about 24 hours.

Nutritional Information:
Calories: 454, Fat:23.9 g, Carbs:50.9 g, Protein:14.6 g, Sugars:14.9 g, Sodium:162 mg

Sunday Morning Waffles

Prep time: 5 mins | Servings: 6

Ingredients:
- 2 egg whites
- ¼ c. sugar
- 2 tsps. Pure vanilla extract
- 1 tbsp. sodium-free baking powder
- 2 tbsps. Canola oil
- 1 2/3 c. unbleached all-purpose flour
- 1 ½ c. low-fat milk

Directions:
1. Spray waffle iron lightly with oil and preheat. Measure the flour, sugar, and baking powder into a mixing bowl and whisk well to combine. Add milk, vanilla, and canola oil to the dry ingredients and mix well. Let rest for 1–2 minutes to thicken.
2. While batter is thickening, place egg whites into another mixing bowl and beat until they form stiff peaks. Once beaten, gently fold whites into the batter.
3. Ladle batter onto hot surface of waffle iron, being careful to avoid the edges. Close waffle iron and bake until golden brown, roughly 4–5 minutes.
4. Remove baked waffle from iron and repeat process with remaining batter, re-oiling waffle iron as necessary. Serve immediately.

Nutritional Information:
Calories: 220, Fat:6 g, Carbs:35 g, Protein:7 g, Sugars:6 g, Sodium:370 mg

Oat Smoothie

Prep time: 5 mins | Servings: 4

Ingredients:
- 2 peeled and sliced bananas
- 2 peeled, seeded and sectioned oranges
- 1 c. crushed ice cubes
- 2/3 c. rolled oats
- 2 c. unsweetened almond milk

Directions:
1. In a high-speed blender, add rolled oats and pulse until finely chopped.
2. Add remaining ingredients and pulse until smooth.
3. Transfer into 4 serving glasses and serve immediately.

Nutritional Information:
Calories: 175, Fat:3 g, Carbs:36.6 g, Protein:3.9 g, Sugars:5 g, Sodium:92 mg

Saturday Morning Pancakes

Prep time: 5 mins | Servings 4

Ingredients:
- 1 tbsp. pure vanilla extract
- ¼ c. sugar
- 1 tbsp. sodium-free baking powder
- 1 tbsp. canola oil
- 1 1/3 c. white whole-wheat flour
- 1 ½ c. low-fat milk
- 1 egg white

Directions:
1. Measure the flour, sugar, and baking powder into a mixing bowl and whisk well to combine.
2. Add the milk, egg white, oil, and vanilla. Mix well and let sit for 1–2 minutes to thicken.
3. Place nonstick griddle or skillet on stove and turn heat to medium-low. Pour batter onto heated griddle. When pancake has bubbled on top and is nicely browned on bottom approximately 2 to 4 minutes, flip over. Brown on second side another 2–3 minutes. If pancakes are browning too quickly, lower heat to low.
4. Repeat process with remaining batter. Serve pancakes warm.

Nutritional Information:
Calories: 266, Fat:5 g, Carbs:46 g, Protein:9 g, Sugars:17 g, Sodium:62 mg

Breakfast Banana Split

Prep time: 10 mins | Servings: 1-2

Ingredients:
- ½ c. canned pineapple titbits
- ½ c. granola cereal
- ½ tsp. honey
- 1 small banana
- ½ c. low fat vanilla yogurt

Directions:
1. Remove the banana and cut it in length and divide them into 2 different bowls.
2. Dust granola over it and save some for the garnishing.
3. Drop yogurt on the paramount and sprinkle with honey and serve it instantly with a bit more granola and pineapple.

Nutritional Information:
Calories: 354.2, Fat:4.1 g, Carbs:74.9 g, Protein:8.7 g, Sugars:23.5 g, Sodium:110.5 mg

Multigrain Hot Cereal

Prep time: 5 mins | Servings: 8

Ingredients:
- ½ c. brown rice
- ¼ tsp. kosher salt
- ½ c. red wheat berries
- 1½ quarts water
- ½ c. pearl barley
- ¼ c. steel cut oats
- 3 tbsps. Quinoa

Directions:
1. Add all ingredients to a saucepan, stir to mix and bring to a boil.
2. Reduce the heat to low and allow to simmer for 45 minutes giving it an occasional stir.
3. The cereal can be refrigerated and reheated for quick breakfasts or snacks throughout the week.

Nutritional Information:
Calories: 118, Fat:1.0 g, Carbs:23.6 g, Protein:4.0 g, Sugars:3 g, Sodium:70 mg

Quinoa Porridge

Prep time: 10 mins | Servings: 6

Ingredients:
- 2 tsps. Vanilla extract
- 2 c. water
- 2 tbsps. Lemon juice
- Salt
- 1 c. raisins
- 2 c. apple juice
- 1 c. quinoa
- 1 tsp. cinnamon

Directions:
1. Wash quinoa thorough by placing in a sieve and rinsing.
2. Allow to drain, and then add quinoa to a saucepan with the two cups of water.
3. Bring to the boil over high heat. Cover pan with lid, lower heat, and simmer until all the water is absorbed, and quinoa is tender. This should take about 15 minutes.
4. Mix in the apple juice, raisins, lemon juice, cinnamon, and salt.
5. Cover the pan and allow to simmer for another 15 minutes.
6. Stir in the vanilla extract and serve immediately.

Nutritional Information:
Calories: 218, Fat:2 g, Carbs:49 g, Protein:5 g, Sugars:2.8 g, Sodium:46 mg

French Toasts Casserole

Prep time: 5 mins | Servings: 2

Ingredients:
- 1 c. slightly beaten egg whites
- 2 tbsps. Applesauce
- 2 cubed whole-wheat bread slices
- 2 tbsps. Chopped almonds
- 2 tsps. Softened unsalted margarine

Directions:
1. In a microwave safe bowl, mix the cubed bread and margarine.
2. Top with egg whites evenly and drizzle with applesauce.
3. Microwave on high for about 1 minute.
4. Remove from microwave and push away the edges of egg whites with a spoon.
5. Microwave for about 1 minute more.
6. Remove from microwave and divide into 2 portions.
7. Serve warm, topped with almonds.

Nutritional Information:
Calories: 207, Fat:7.9 g, Carbs:15.5 g, Protein:18.2 g, Sugars:25 g, Sodium:257 mg

Delicious Omelet

Prep time: 10 mins | Servings: 2

Ingredients:
- ¼ c. low-fat Mexican cheese
- 2 tbsps. Water
- 1 tsp. organic olive oil
- ¼ tsp. black pepper
- 2 eggs
- ¼ c. chunky salsa

Directions:
1. In a bowl, combine the eggs with all the water, cheese, salsa and pepper and whisk well.
2. Heat up a pan with all the oil over medium-high heat, add the eggs mix, spread in for the pan, cook for 3 minutes, flip, cook for 3 more minutes, divide between plates and serve enjoying.
3. Enjoy!

Nutritional Information:
Calories: 221, Fat:4 g, Carbs:13 g, Protein:7 g, Sugars:4 g, Sodium:700 mg

Chicken Breakfast Burrito

Prep time: 5 mins | Servings: 2

Ingredients:
- 2 tbsps. Italian salad dressing
- 1 whole wheat tortilla
- 1 sliced pear
- 4 oz. cooked skinless chicken
- 1 c. fresh spinach

Directions:
1. Slice the chicken into small bite-sized pieces and arrange them on the tortilla.
2. Cover the meat with spinach and arrange the pear slices on top.
3. Drizzle with Italian salad dressing.
4. Wrap the tortilla around all the ingredients until it's a snug burrito.

Nutritional Information:
Calories: 246, Fat:10.3 g, Carbs:23.6 g, Protein:15.6 g, Sugars:3 g, Sodium:850 mg

Breakfast Sausage Crepe Filling

Prep time: 15 mins | Servings: 2

Ingredients:
- 8 crepes
- 8 small cooked sausages

Directions:
1. Cook the sausage according to the directions on the package.
2. Stuff the crepe with two sausages.
3. Serve immediately.

Nutritional Information:
Calories: 60, Fat:0.2 g, Carbs:75 g, Protein:1.7 g, Sugars:12 g, Sodium:137 mg

Banana Bread

Prep time: 15 mins | Servings: 20

Ingredients:
- 2 ¼ g ground cinnamon
- 2 whole eggs
- 85 g coconut sugar
- 11 ¼ g salt
- 2 ¼ g baking soda
- 455 g All-purpose flour
- 75 g softened butter
- 3 mashed ripe bananas
- 1 ¼ g baking powder

Directions:
1. Preheat the oven to 400 °F and grease two small loaf pans with a touch of butter and set aside.
2. In two separate dishes mix your dry and wet ingredients. Start by putting the softened butter, eggs, and mashed bananas into a bowl and slowly mix in the coconut sugar, until smooth.
3. In another bowl, shift your flour, salt, baking soda, baking powder, and a touch of cinnamon if you like the flavor. You can also use powdered cardamom for a slightly more aromatic flavor.
4. Combine the ingredients, and either blend or mix by hand, whichever you prefer. Add in any extra ingredients you want to use, pour the dough into the prepped pans, and put them in to bake for 20 minutes exactly.
5. Once baked, use a knife or a toothpick to test if the loaves have cooked through, and you're all done!
6. You can easily slice and store the bread for later, so don't forget to have a container handy to store your fresh banana bread for the next week!

Nutritional Information:
Calories: 133, Fat:3.4 g, Carbs:11 g, Protein:4.3 g, Sugars:7.5 g, Sodium:205 mg

Spinach Muffins

Prep time: 10 mins | Servings: 6

Ingredients:
- 4 oz. spinach
- 2 oz. chopped prosciutto
- ½ c. non-fat milk
- Cooking spray
- 6 eggs
- 1 c. crumbled low-fat cheese
- ½ c. chopped roasted red pepper

Directions:
1. In a bowl, combine the eggs using the milk, cheese, spinach, red pepper and prosciutto and whisk well.
2. Grease a muffin tray with cooking spray, divide the muffin mix, introduce within the oven and bake at 350 °F for around 30 minutes.
3. Divide between plates and serve enjoying.
4. Enjoy!

Nutritional Information:
Calories: 155, Fat:10 g, Carbs:4 g, Protein:10 g, Sugars:0.6 g, Sodium:195 mg

Chia Seeds Breakfast Mix

Prep time: 8 hours | Servings: 4

Ingredients:
- 1 tsp. grated lemon zest
- 4 tbsps. Chia seeds
- 1 c. blueberries
- 4 tbsps. Coconut sugar
- 2 c. old-fashioned oats
- 3 c. coconut milk

Directions:
1. In a bowl, combine the oats with chia seeds, sugar, milk, lemon zest and blueberries, stir, and divide into cups whilst within the fridge for 8 hours.
2. Serve enjoying.
3. Enjoy!

Nutritional Information:
Calories: 283, Fat:12 g, Carbs:13 g, Protein:8 g, Sugars:3.6 g, Sodium:8 mg

Breakfast Fruits Bowls

Prep time: 10 mins | Servings: 2

Ingredients:
- 1 c. chopped pineapple
- 1 sliced banana
- 1 c. chopped mango
- 1 c. almond milk

Directions:
1. In a bowl, combine the mango with all the current banana, pineapple and almond milk, stir, divide into smaller bowls and serve each day.
2. Enjoy!

Nutritional Information:
Calories: 182, Fat:2 g, Carbs:12 g, Protein:6 g, Sugars:6 g, Sodium:110 mg

Easy Omelet Waffles

Prep time: 10 mins | Servings: 2

Ingredients:
- Cooking spray
- 2 tbsps. Chopped parsley
- ¼ tsp. black pepper
- ¼ c. shredded low-fat cheddar
- 4 eggs
- 2 tbsps. Chopped ham

Directions:
1. In a bowl, combine the eggs with pepper, ham, cheese and parsley and whisk effectively.
2. Grease your waffle iron with cooking spray, add the eggs mix, cook for 4-5 minutes, divide the waffles between plates and serve them for breakfast.
3. Enjoy!

Nutritional Information:
Calories: 211, Fat:3 g, Carbs:14 g, Protein:8 g, Sugars:1 g, Sodium:1000 mg

Pesto Omelet

Prep time: 10 mins | Servings: 2

Ingredients:
- Chopped cherry tomatoes
- 4 eggs
- 3 tbsps. Pistachio pesto
- 2 tsps. Essential organic olive oil
- ¼ tsp. black pepper

Directions:

1. In a bowl, combine the eggs with cherry tomatoes, black pepper and pistachio pesto and whisk well.
2. Heat up a pan while using oil over medium-high heat, add eggs mix, spread in the pan, cook for 3 minutes, flip, cook for 3 minutes more, divide between 2 plates and serve enjoying.
3. Enjoy!

Nutritional Information:
Calories: 199, Fat:2 g, Carbs:14 g, Protein:7 g, Sugars:16 g, Sodium:600 mg

Strawberry Sandwich

Prep time: 10 mins | Servings: 4

Ingredients:
- 1 tbsp. stevia
- 2 c. sliced strawberries
- 1 tsp. grated lemon zest
- 8 oz. soft low-fat cream cheese, soft
- 4 halved and toasted wheat grains English muffins

Directions:
1. In the meat processor, combine the cream cheese with the stevia and lemon zest and pulse well.
2. Spread 1 tablespoon with this mix on 1 muffin half and top with many of the sliced strawberries.
3. Repeat with all the rest from the muffin halves and serve enjoying.
4. Enjoy!

Nutritional Information:
Calories: 211, Fat:3 g, Carbs:8 g, Protein:4 g, Sugars:8 g, Sodium:70 mg

Irish Brown Bread

Prep time: 10 mins | Servings: 4

Ingredients:
- 4 tsps. Baking soda
- 3 c. all-purpose flour
- 4 c. low fat buttermilk
- 2 beaten eggs
- ½ tsp. salt
- 4 c. whole wheat flour
- 1 c. wheat germ

Directions:
1. Mix together all the dry Ingredients in a large bowl.
2. Add buttermilk and egg and mix until it forms a dough.
3. Transfer the dough onto a floured work area and knead gently.
4. Place on a nonstick baking sheet and form a large round. Cut an "X" shape in the center of the round, about 1/2 inch deep.
5. Bake in a preheated oven at 400 degree F for about 25-30 minutes or until the bread splits apart at the X cut.
6. When done, remove and place on a wire rack and cool completely.
7. Slice and serve.

Nutritional Information:
Calories: 92.1, Fat:1.2 g, Carbs:17.6 g, Protein:3.7 g, Sugars:2 g, Sodium:244 mg

Fresh Fruit Crunch

Prep time: 5 mins | Servings: 2

Ingredients:
- 2 tbsps. Toasted coconut
- 1 c. low fat vanilla yogurt
- ¼ c. low fat granola
- 2 c. mixed fresh fruits
- 1 tbsp. honey

Directions:
1. Divide the fruits into 2 tall glasses.
2. Divide the yogurt and spoon over the fruits.

3. Drizzle honey on top.
4. Top with granola and coconut. Refrigerate until chilled.
5. Serve cold.

Nutritional Information:
Calories: 358, Fat:5.4 g, Carbs:61.8 g, Protein:8.3 g, Sugars:6 g, Sodium:40 mg

Apple and Quinoa Breakfast Bake

Prep time: 10 mins | Servings: 6

Ingredients:
- 1 tsp. cinnamon powder
- 2 cored, peeled and chopped apples
- ¼ tsp. extra virgin organic olive oil
- ½ c. almond milk
- 2 tsps. Coconut sugar
- 1 c. cooked quinoa

Directions:
1. Grease a ramekin with all the current oil, add quinoa, apples, sugar, cinnamon and almond milk, stir, introduce inside oven, bake at 350 °F for 10 minutes, divide into bowls and serve.
2. Enjoy!

Nutritional Information:
Calories: 199, Fat:2 g, Carbs:14 g, Protein:8 g, Sugars:25 g, Sodium:170 mg

Banana and Pear Breakfast Salad

Prep time: 10 mins | Servings: 2

Ingredients:
- 1 cored and cubed Asian pear
- ½ tsp. cinnamon powder
- 1 peeled and sliced banana
- 2 oz. toasted pepitas
- ½ lime juice

Directions:
1. In a bowl, combine the banana using the pear, lime juice, cinnamon and pepitas, toss, divide between small plates and serve enjoying.
2. Enjoy!

Nutritional Information:
Calories: 188, Fat:2 g, Carbs:5 g, Protein:7 g, Sugars:10 g, Sodium:300 mg

Apple Cinnamon Crisp

Prep time: 10 mins | Servings: 4

Ingredients:
- 1 tsp. cinnamon
- 1 c. brown sugar
- 3 lbs. Granny Smith apples
- 2 tbsps. All-purpose flour
- 1 stick butter
- 1 c. oatmeal
- 1 tbsp. granulated sugar

Directions:
1. Peel and core the apples, slice thinly.
2. Mix granulated sugar with flour and add the apples. Toss to coat.
3. Put apples into the bottom of a 5-6 quart crock pot.
4. Combine brown sugar with oatmeal and butter. Mix until mixture is crumbly.
5. Sprinkle oatmeal mixture on top of the apples.
6. Cook apples fully on high heat.

Nutritional Information:
Calories: 549, Fat:27 g, Carbs:71 g, Protein:6 g, Sugars:43 g, Sodium:430 mg

Peanut Butter & Blueberry Parfait

Prep time: 5 mins | Servings: 2

Ingredients:
- ½ c. chopped almonds
- 1 tbsp. unsweetened peanut butter
- ½ tsp. cinnamon
- 1 tsp. honey
- 1 c. low fat vanilla yogurt
- 1 c. blueberries

Directions:
1. Combine the yogurt and peanut butter. Mix until blended and set aside.
2. Combine the blueberries, almonds, honey, and cinnamon. Toss to mix.
3. In two separate serving glasses, alternate layers of the yogurt and blueberry mixture until all ingredients have been used.
4. Serve immediately or chill until ready to serve.

Nutritional Information:
Calories: 194.1, Fat:5.0 g, Carbs:31.1 g, Protein:6.8 g, Sugars:8.4 g, Sodium:48 mg

Quinoa Quiche

Prep time: 10 mins | Servings: 4

Ingredients:
- 1 c. fat-free ricotta cheese
- 2/3 c. grated low-fat parmesan
- 3 oz. chopped spinach
- 1 ½ tsps. Garlic powder
- 1 c. cooked quinoa
- 3 eggs

Directions:
1. In a bowl, combine the quinoa while using spinach, ricotta, eggs, garlic powder and parmesan, whisk well, pour into a lined pie pan, introduce inside oven and bake at 355 °F for 45 minutes.
2. Cool the quiche down, slice and serve enjoying.
3. Enjoy!

Nutritional Information:
Calories: 201, Fat:2 g, Carbs:12 g, Protein:7 g, Sugars:0 g, Sodium:130 mg

Sweet Rosemary Oats

Prep time: 5 mins | Servings: 2

Ingredients:
- 2 tbsps. Chopped fresh rosemary
- 1 tbsp. honey
- ½ c. chopped walnuts
- Fresh strawberries
- 2 c. low fat milk
- 2 c. old fashioned oats
- 1 tsp. ground pink peppercorns

Directions:
1. Combine the oats, walnuts, rosemary, and pink pepper in a bowl. Toss to mix and place in a mason jar or other lidded container.
2. Combine the milk and honey and pour over the oat mixture.
3. Cover and refrigerate for 12 hours, or overnight.
4. Warm for 1-2 minutes in the microwave before serving.
5. Top with fresh strawberries, if desired

Nutritional Information:
Calories: 305.3, Fat:13.1 g, Carbs:39.5 g, Protein:11.4 g, Sugars:1 g, Sodium:520 mg

Egg Parsley Omelet

Prep time: 15 mins | Servings: 5-6

Ingredients:
- ¼ tsp. black pepper
- 2 tsps. Olive oil
- 2 tbsps. Chopped parsley
- 1 tbsp. shredded low-fat cheddar cheese
- 6 whisked eggs
- 2 tbsps. almond milk

Directions:
1. In a bowl of medium-large size, thoroughly stir the eggs, milk, pepper, parsley, and cheese.
2. Heat some olive oil in a pan over medium flame; add the eggs mix, spreading evenly along the pan.
3. Cook for 2-3 minutes, flip, cook for 3 minutes more.
4. Serve warm.

Nutritional Information:
Calories: 238, Fat:20.6 g, Carbs:2.7 g, Protein:11.9 g, Sugars:0.5 g, Sodium:804.2 mg

Quinoa Breakfast Bars

Prep time: 2 hours | Servings: 6

Ingredients:
- 1/3 c. flaked coconut
- ½ tsp. cinnamon powder
- 2 tbsps. Coconut sugar
- 2 tbsps. Unsweetened chocolate chips
- ½ c. fat-free peanut butter
- 1 tsp. vanilla flavoring
- 1 c. quinoa flakes

Directions:
1. In a large bowl, combine the peanut butter with sugar, vanilla, cinnamon, quinoa, coconut and chocolate chips, stir well, spread about the bottom of the lined baking sheet, press well, cut in 6 bars, keep inside fridge for just two hours, divide between plates and serve.
2. Enjoy!

Nutritional Information:
Calories: 182, Fat:4 g, Carbs:13 g, Protein:11 g, Sugars:14.8 g, Sodium:69 mg

Granola Breakfast Pops

Prep time: 5 mins | Servings: 4-6

Ingredients:
- ½ c. chopped fresh pineapple
- ½ c. chopped mango
- 2 c. low fat vanilla yogurt
- ¼ c. sugar free granola
- ½ c. chopped strawberries

Directions:
1. Combine the yogurt, strawberries, pineapple, and mango in a bowl. Mix well.
2. Transfer the yogurt mixture to ice pop molds and then sprinkle a little bit of granola into each.
3. Place in the freezer and freeze for several hours or overnight.

Nutritional Information:
Calories: 133.8, Fat:1.4 g, Carbs:25.5 g, Protein:5.1 g, Sugars:13 g, Sodium:10 mg

Cinnamon Breakfast Quinoa

Prep time: 10 mins | Servings: 2

Ingredients:
- ¾ c. water
- ½ c. rinsed and drained quinoa
- Milk
- 2 tbsps. Chopped walnuts
- Honey
- 1/8 tsp. salt
- 1 stick cinnamon

Directions:
1. Place a heavy bottomed saucepan over a medium heat. Add quinoa, water, salt and cinnamon. Mix well and bring to a boil.
2. Lower the heat, cover and simmer until all the water is absorbed.
3. Remove from the heat. Do not uncover for 5 minutes.
4. Fluff the cooked quinoa with a fork and discard the cinnamon stick.

5. Divide the quinoa into individual serving bowls. Pour milk over the quinoa.
6. Drizzle honey over the quinoa, sprinkle walnuts on top and serve.

Nutritional Information:
Calories: 229.3, Fat:3.2 g, Carbs:35.6 g, Protein:6.1 g, Sugars:8 g, Sodium:69 mg

Cinnamon Walnut Breakfast Parfait

Prep time: 10 mins | Servings: 2

Ingredients:
- ¼ tsp. cinnamon
- 1 tsp. chia seeds
- ½ c. chopped walnuts
- 1 c. low fat vanilla yogurt
- 1 c. chopped granny smith apples
- 1 tsp. honey

Directions:
1. In a bowl, combine the yogurt and chia seeds. Set aside.
2. In another bowl, combine the apples, walnuts, honey, and cinnamon. Mix well.
3. In two separate serving glasses, alternate layers of apple walnut mixture and yogurt until all ingredients have been used.
4. Serve immediately or chill before serving.

Nutritional Information:
Calories: 364.2, Fat:23.4 g, Carbs:34.6 g, Protein:10.7 g, Sugars:6 g, Sodium:85 mg

Breakfast Taco

Prep time: 25 mins | Servings: 5

Ingredients:
- ¼ c. sliced bell peppers
- 3 warm tortillas
- 1 tsp. butter
- 3 portions lean meat
- Pepper and salt
- 4 large eggs
- 1 c. organic shredded cheese

Directions:
1. Preheat oven to 300°F. Wrap the tortillas in foil. Place in the oven. Heat for 5 minutes.
2. In a large skillet, cook the meat choice.
3. In a bowl, crack the eggs and mix. Add salt and pepper.
4. In another skillet, melt the butter. Cook the scrambled eggs.
5. Assemble the taco with scrambled egg, meat, bell pepper, cheese.
6. Serve immediately.

Nutritional Information:
Calories: 77, Fat:0.1 g, Carbs:40 g, Protein:0.6 g, Sugars:1 g, Sodium:300 mg

Egg Spinach Breakfast Muffins

Prep time: 40 mins | Servings: 6

Ingredients:
- 2 oz. chopped prosciutto
- 4 oz. chopped spinach
- Cooking spray
- ½ c. chopped roasted red pepper
- 1 c. crumbled low-fat cheese
- 6 eggs
- ½ c. skim milk

Directions:
1. In a mixing bowl, thoroughly mix the eggs, milk, cheese, spinach, red pepper, and prosciutto.
2. Grease the muffin tins with some cooking spray.
3. Pour the muffin mix in the tins.
4. Bake in the preheated oven at 350 °F for 25-30 minutes.
5. Serve warm.

Nutritional Information:
Calories: 98.9, Fat:6.7 g, Carbs:0.9 g, Protein:8.0 g, Sugars:1.5 g, Sodium:79 mg

Whole Grain Toast with Fruited Ricotta Spread

Prep time: 10 mins | Servings: 4

Ingredients:
- 2 tsps. Honey
- 1 c. low fat ricotta cheese
- ½ c. finely diced peaches
- 1 tsp. orange zest
- ¼ c. sliced almonds
- 4 toasted whole grain bread slices
- 1 tbsp. fresh chopped mint

Directions:
1. In a bowl, combine the ricotta cheese, orange zest, honey, mint, and peaches. Blend well.
2. Spread evenly on each piece of whole wheat toast and top with sliced almonds and additional fresh fruit, if desired.

Nutritional Information:
Calories: 196.1, Fat:8.9 g, Carbs:20.0 g, Protein:12.4 g, Sugars:7 g, Sodium:190 mg

Cherries Oatmeal

Prep time: 10 mins | Servings: 6

Ingredients:
- 2 c. pitted and sliced cherries
- 6 c. water
- 1 tsp. cinnamon powder
- 1 c. almond milk
- 2 c. old-fashioned oats
- 1 tsp. vanilla flavor

Directions:
1. In a little pot, combine the oats while using the water, milk, cinnamon, vanilla and cherries, toss, bring to a simmer over medium-high heat, cook for quarter-hour, divide into bowls and serve in the morning.
2. Enjoy!

Nutritional Information:
Calories 180, Fat 4g, Fiber 4g, Carbs 9g, Protein 7g, Sodium 98mg, Sugars 14g

Strawberry Chia Breakfast Pudding

Prep time: 5 mins | Servings: 4

Ingredients:
- 1 tbsp. honey
- 3 c. chopped strawberries
- 1 tsp. pure vanilla extract
- 2 c. unsweetened coconut milk
- ½ c. chia seeds

Directions:
1. Combine the coconut milk and strawberries in a blender and puree until smooth.
2. Add the chia seeds, vanilla extract, and honey. Stir well.
3. Cover and refrigerate at least 6 hours or overnight.

Nutritional Information:
Calories:314.8 , Fat:25.0 g, Carbs:22.1 g, Protein:4.5 g, Sugars:7.4 g, Sodium:46 mg

Banana Nutty Oats

Prep time: 30 mins. | Servings: 4

Ingredients:
- 2 c. water
- 2 tbsps. Chia seeds
- ¼ c. chopped walnuts
- 1 tsp. vanilla extract
- 2 peeled and mashed bananas
- 1 c. almond milk
- 1 c. steel-cut oats

Directions:

1. In a cooking pot, mix the water with the oats, milk, walnuts, chia seeds, bananas, and vanilla.
2. Combine well and boil the mix over medium flame.
3. Simmer for 15 minutes, stirring frequently.
4. Transfer to your serving bowls and serve warm.

Nutritional Information:
Calories: 425, Fat:17.5 g, Carbs:62.5 g, Protein:12.5 g, Sugars:22.5 g, Sodium:212.2 mg

Breakfast Apple and Raisin Oatmeal

Prep time: 10 mins | Servings: 2

Ingredients:
- 1 c. old fashioned oats
- 2 tbsps. Honey
- ¼ c. raisins
- ½ tsp. ground cinnamon
- 2 drops vanilla essence
- 2 c. milk low-fat milk
- 1 tbsp. light butter
- 1 c. chopped apples

Directions:
1. Use a Crock Pot Liner or spray the inside of a 5-quart slow cooker with non-stick cooking spray
2. Combine all ingredients to the slow cooker and stir well to combine.
3. Cover and cook on LOW overnight, ideally no more than 6 hours or it will dry out.
4. Stir well in the morning before serving.

Nutritional Information:
Calories: 240, Fat:3.9 g, Carbs:49 g, Protein:4.6 g, Sugars:38 g, Sodium:62 mg

Fast Punch

Prep time: 5 mins | Servings: 6

Ingredients:
- 4 tbsps. Lemon juice
- 2 c. peeled citrus fruits
- 1 c. ice
- 8 oz. cranberry juice
- 1 ½ c. chopped pineapple

Directions:
1. Place all ingredients in a food blender.
2. Puree until smooth.
3. Serve immediately.

Nutritional Information:
Calories: 116.6, Fat:0 g, Carbs:29.6 g, Protein:0 g, Sugars:28 g, Sodium:94.2 mg

Chocolate Covered Banana Quinoa

Prep time: 5 mins | Servings: 4

Ingredients:
- 1 tbsp. honey
- ¼ c. dark chocolate shavings
- 2 tsps. Dark cocoa powder
- 1 c. sliced banana
- 2 c. low fat milk
- 1 c. uncooked quinoa

Directions:
1. In a saucepan, combine the milk with the dark cocoa powder and honey. Heat over medium to medium high heat until mixture bubbles, stirring frequently.
2. Add the quinoa and reduce heat to low. Cover and simmer for 15-20 minutes, or until most of the liquid is absorbed and grain is tender.
3. Serve warm garnished with sliced banana and chocolate shavings, if desired.

Nutritional Information:
Calories: 256.5, Fat:4.4 g, Carbs:49.4 g, Protein:7.4 g, Sugars:5 g, Sodium:155 mg

Chapter 3 Vegetarian and Vegan

Baked Potatoes and "BBQ" Lentils

Prep time: 5 mins | Servings: 4

Ingredients:
- 2 sliced large baked potatoes
- 1 c. dry brown lentils
- 2 tsps. molasses
- 1 chopped small onion
- 2 tsps. liquid smoke
- 3 c. water
- ½ c. organic ketchup

Directions:
1. Add water, onion and lentils to the pot
2. Lock up the lid and cook on HIGH pressure for 10 minutes
3. Release the pressure naturally
4. Add ketchup, liquid smoke and molasses to the lentil
5. Sauté for 5 minutes
6. Serve over baked potatoes and enjoy!

Nutritional Information:
Calories: 140, Fat:4 g, Carbs:24 g, Protein:5 g, Sugars:606 g, Sodium:18 mg

Orange Juice Smoothie

Prep time: 5 mins | Servings: 2

Ingredients:
- ¼ c. frozen orange juice concentrate
- ¾ c. fat-free milk
- 1 c. fat-free vanilla frozen yogurt

Directions:
1. Add the ingredients to a blender and pulse until they're smooth.
2. Pour them into frosted glasses and serve.

Nutritional Information:
Calories: 180, Fat:0 g, Carbs:38 g, Protein:7 g, Sugars:20 g, Sodium:5 mg

Superb Lemon Roasted Artichokes

Prep time: 10 mins | Servings: 2

Ingredients
- 2 peeled and sliced garlic cloves
- 3 lemon pieces
- Black pepper
- 2 artichoke pieces
- 3 tbsps. olive oil
- Sea flavored vinegar

Directions:
1. Wash your artichokes well and dip them in water and cut the stem to about ½ inch long
2. Trim the thorny tips and outer leaves and rub the chokes with lemon
3. Poke garlic slivers between the choke leaves and place a trivet basket in the Instant Pot ten add artichokes
4. Lock up the lid and cook on high pressure for 7 minutes
5. Release the pressure naturally over 10 minutes
6. Transfer the artichokes to cutting board and allow them to cool then cut half lengthwise and cut the purple white center
7. Pre-heat your oven to 400 degree Fahrenheit
8. Take a bowl and mix 1 and ½ lemon and olive oil
9. Pour over the choke halves and sprinkle flavored vinegar and pepper
10. Place an iron skillet in your oven and heat it up for 5 minutes
11. Add a few teaspoon of oil and place the marinated artichoke halves in the skillet
12. Brush with lemon and olive oil mixture

13. Cut third lemon in quarter and nestle them between the halves
14. Roast for 20-25 minutes until the chokes are browned
15. Serve and enjoy!

Nutritional Information:
Calories: 263, Fat:16 g, Carbs:8 g, Protein:23 g, Sugars:128 g, Sodium:0.4 mg

Chocolate Aquafaba Mousse

Prep time: 20 mins | Servings: 4-6

Ingredients:
- 1 tsp. pure vanilla extract
- 15 oz. unsalted chickpeas
- Fresh raspberries
- ¼ tsp. tartar cream
- 6 oz. dairy-free dark chocolate
- 2 tbsps. coconut sugar
- ¼ tsp. sea salt

Directions:
1. Chop dark chocolate into coarse bits and place the chocolate into a glass bowl over boiling water on the stovetop or in a double boiler.
2. Melt the chocolate gently, stirring until completely melted.
3. Remove the melted chocolate from the heat and pour the chocolate into a large bowl.
4. Drain the chickpeas, reserving the brine (aquafaba), and store the chickpeas for another recipe like hummus.
5. Add in the aquafaba along with cream of tartar.
6. Mix on high speed using an electric hand mixer for 7-10 minutes, or until soft peaks begin to form.
7. Add in the salt, vanilla extract, and coconut sugar and beat the mixture until well mixed.
8. Add half of the melted chocolate to the whipped aquafaba and fold it in until incorporated.
9. Fold in the remaining aquafaba until smooth and well combined to form the mousse.
10. Gently spoon the chocolate mousse into glasses, ramekins or small mason jars.
11. Cover with cling film and chill for at least 3 hours.
12. Sprinkle he mousse with raspberries and serve.

Nutritional Information:
Calories: 280, Fat:13.8 g, Carbs:34.7 g, Protein:3.9 g, Sugars:22 g, Sodium:242 mg

Hearty Baby Carrots

Prep time: 5 mins | Servings: 4

Ingredients:
- 1 tbsp. chopped fresh mint
- 1 c. water
- Sea flavored vinegar
- 1 lb. baby carrots
- 1 tbsp. clarified ghee

Directions:
1. Place a steamer rack on top of your pot and add the carrots
2. Add water
3. Lock up the lid and cook at HIGH pressure for 2 minutes
4. Do a quick release
5. Pass the carrots through a strainer and drain them
6. Wipe the insert clean
7. Return the insert to the pot and set the pot to Sauté mode
8. Add clarified butter and allow it to melt
9. Add mint and sauté for 30 seconds
10. Add carrots to the insert and sauté well
11. Remove them and sprinkle with bit of flavored vinegar on top
12. Enjoy!

Nutritional Information:
Calories: 131, Fat:10 g, Carbs:11 g, Protein:1 g, Sugars:5 g, Sodium:190 mg

Sensitive Steamed Artichokes

Prep time: 5 mins | Servings: 4

Ingredients:
- 1 halved lemon
- ¼ tsp. paprika
- 2 tbsps. Homemade Whole30 mayo
- 2 medium artichokes
- 1 tsp. Dijon mustard

Directions:
1. Wash the artichokes and remove the damaged outer leaves
2. Trim the spines and cut off upper edge
3. Wipe the cur edges with lemon half
4. Slice the stem and peel the stem
5. Chop it up and keep them on the side
6. Add a cup of water to the pot and place a steamer basket inside
7. Transfer the artichokes to the steamer basket and a squeeze of lemon
8. Lock up the lid and cook on HIGH pressure for 10 minutes
9. Release the pressure naturally
10. Enjoy

Nutritional Information:
Calories: 77, Fat:5 g, Carbs:0 g, Protein:2 g, Sugars:1.3 g, Sodium:121 mg

Minted Peas Feta Rice

Prep time: 15 mins | Servings: 2

Ingredients:
- 1 ¼ c. vegetable broth
- ¾ c. brown rice
- ¼ c. finely crumbled feta cheese
- ¾ c. sliced scallions
- 1 ½ c. frozen peas
- Freshly ground pepper
- ¼ c. sliced fresh mint

Directions:
1. Boil broth in a saucepan over medium heat.
2. Add rice and bring it to a simmer. Cook for 4 minutes.
3. Stir in peas and cook for 6 minutes.
4. Turn off the heat then add feta, mint, scallions, and pepper.
5. Serve warm.

Nutritional Information:
Calories: 28.1, Fat:18.2 g, Carbs:10.3 g, Protein:8.8 g, Sugars:2.2 g, Sodium:216 mg

Rhubarb and Strawberry Compote

Prep time: 10 mins | Servings: 4

Ingredients:
- 3 tbsps. Date paste
- ½ c. water
- Fresh mint
- 2 lbs. rhubarb
- 1 lb. strawberries

Directions:
1. Peel the rhubarb using a paring knife and chop it up ½ inch pieces
2. Add the chopped up rhubarb to your pot alongside water
3. Lock up the lid and cook on HIGH pressure for 10 minutes
4. Stem and quarter your strawberries and keep them on the side
5. Add the strawberries and date paste, give it a nice stir
6. Lock up the lid and cook on HIGH pressure for 20 minutes
7. Release the pressure naturally and enjoy the compote!

Nutritional Information:
Calories: 41.1, Fat:2.1 g, Carbs:5.5 g, Protein:1.4 g, Sugars:12 g, Sodium:2.4 mg

Zucchini Cakes

Prep time: 10 mins | Servings: 4

Ingredients:
- Freshly ground black pepper
- 1 finely diced red onion
- 2 tsps. Salt
- 1 egg white
- Homemade horseradish sauce
- 1 shredded medium zucchini
- ¾ c. salt-free bread crumbs

Directions:
1. Preheat oven to 400°F. Spray a baking sheet lightly with oil and set aside.
2. Press shredded zucchini gently between paper towels to remove excess liquid.
3. In a large bowl, combine zucchini, onion, egg white, bread crumbs, seasoning, and black pepper. Mix well.
4. Shape mixture into patties and place on the prepared baking sheet.
5. Place baking sheet on middle rack in oven and bake for 10 minutes. Gently flip patties and return to oven to bake for another 10 minutes.
6. Remove from oven and serve immediately.

Nutritional Information:
Calories: 94, Fat:1 g, Carbs:19 g, Protein:4 g, Sugars:31 g, Sodium:161 mg

Fresh Fruit Smoothie

Prep time: 5 mins | Servings: 4

Ingredients:
- 1 tbsp. honey
- ½ c. cantaloupe
- 1 c. water
- 1 c. fresh strawberries
- 1 c. fresh pineapple
- 2 orange juice

Directions:
1. Remove the rind from the melon and pineapple. Cut them into chunks and remove the stems from the strawberries.
2. Put everything in a blender and serve.

Nutritional Information:
Calories: 72, Fat:1 g, Carbs:17 g, Protein:1 g, Sugars:1 g, Sodium:42 mg

Popovers

Prep time: 5 mins | Servings: 6

Ingredients:
- 4 egg whites
- 1 c. All-purpose flour
- 1 c. fat-free milk
- ¼ tsp. salt

Directions:
1. Preheat your oven to 425 °F.
2. Coat a six cup metal or glass muffin mold with cooking spray and heat the mold in the oven for two minutes.
3. In a bowl, add the flour, milk, salt, and egg whites. Use a mixer to beat until it's smooth.
4. Fill the heated molds two-thirds of the way full.
5. Bake until the muffins are golden brown and puffy, around half an hour. Serve.

Nutritional Information:
Calories: 101, Fat:0 g, Carbs:18 g, Protein:6 g, Sugars:2 g, Sodium:125 mg

Broccoli, Garlic, and Rigatoni

Prep time: 10 mins | Servings: 2

Ingredients:
- 2 tsps. Minced garlic
- 2 c. Broccoli florets
- Freshly ground black pepper
- 2 tbsps. Parmesan cheese
- 1/3 lb. Rigatoni noodles
- 2 tsps. Olive oil

Directions:
1. Fill a pot three-quarters of the way full with water and bring it to a boil. Add the rigatoni and cook until it is firm, around twelve minutes. Drain it thoroughly.
2. As the pasta cooks, bring an inch of water to a boil and put a steamer basket over the top. Add the broccoli and steam for ten minutes.
3. In a bowl, mix together the pasta and broccoli. Toss with the cheese, oil, and garlic.
4. Season to taste and serve.

Nutritional Information:
Calories: 355, Fat:7 g, Carbs:63 g, Protein:14 g, Sugars:4 g, Sodium:600 mg

Vegan Rice Pudding

Prep time: 5 mins | Servings: 8

Ingredients:
- ½ tsp. ground cinnamon
- 1 c. rinsed basmati
- 1/8 tsp. ground cardamom
- ¼ c. sugar
- 1/8 tsp. pure almond extract
- 1 quart vanilla nondairy milk
- 1 tsp. pure vanilla extract

Directions:
1. Measure all of the ingredients into a saucepan and stir well to combine. Bring to a boil over medium-high heat.
2. Once boiling, reduce heat to low and simmer, stirring very frequently, about 15–20 minutes.
3. Remove from heat and cool. Serve sprinkled with additional ground cinnamon if desired.

Nutritional Information:
Calories: 148, Fat:2 g, Carbs:26 g, Protein:4 g, Sugars:35 g, Sodium:150 mg

Cinnamon-scented Quinoa

Prep time: 5 mins | Servings: 4

Ingredients:
- Chopped walnuts
- 1 ½ c. water
- Maple syrup
- 2 cinnamon sticks
- 1 c. quinoa

Directions:
1. Add the quinoa to a bowl and wash it in several changes of water until the water is clear. When washing quinoa, rub grains and allow them to settle before you pour off the water.
2. Use a large fine-mesh sieve to drain the quinoa. Prepare your pressure cooker with a trivet and steaming basket. Place the quinoa and the cinnamon sticks in the basket and pour the water.
3. Close and lock the lid. Cook at high pressure for 6 minutes. When the cooking time is up, release the pressure using the quick release method.
4. Fluff the quinoa with a fork and remove the cinnamon sticks. Divide the cooked quinoa among serving bowls and top with maple syrup and chopped walnuts.

Nutritional Information:
Calories: 160, Fat:3 g, Carbs:28 g, Protein:6 g, Sugars:19 g, Sodium:40 mg

Green Vegetable Smoothie

Prep time: 5 mins | Servings: 4

Ingredients:
- 1 c. cold water
- ½ c. strawberries
- 2 oz. baby spinach
- 1 lemon juice
- 1 tbsp. fresh mint
- 1 banana
- ½ c. blueberries

Directions:
1. Put all the ingredients in a juicer or blender and puree.

Nutritional Information:
Calories: 52, Fat:2 g, Carbs:12 g, Protein:1 g, Sugars:18 g, Sodium:36 mg

Garlic Lovers Hummus

Prep time: 2 mins | Servings: 12

Ingredients:
- 3 tbsps. Freshly squeezed lemon juice
- All-purpose salt-free seasoning
- 3 tbsps. Sesame tahini
- 4 garlic cloves
- 15 oz. no-salt-added garbanzo beans
- 2 tbsps. Olive oil

Directions:
1. Drain garbanzo beans and rinse well.
2. Place all the ingredients in a food processor and pulse until smooth.
3. Serve immediately or cover and refrigerate until serving.

Nutritional Information:
Calories: 103, Fat:5 g, Carbs:11 g, Protein:4 g, Sugars:2 g, Sodium:88 mg

Spinach and Kale Mix

Prep time: 5 mins | Servings: 4

Ingredients:
- 2 chopped shallots
- 1 c. no-salt-added and chopped canned tomatoes
- 2 c. baby spinach
- 2 minced garlic cloves
- 5 c. torn kale
- 1 tbsp. olive oil

Directions:
1. Heat up a pan with the oil over medium-high heat, add the shallots, stir and sauté for 5 minutes.
2. Add the spinach, kale and the other ingredients, toss, cook for 10 minutes more, divide between plates and serve.

Nutritional Information:
Calories: 89, Fat:3.7 g, Carbs:12.4 g, Protein:3.6 g, Sugars:0 g, Sodium:50 mg

Apples and Cabbage Mix

Prep time: 5 mins | Servings: 4

Ingredients:
- 2 cored and cubed green apples
- 2 tbsps. balsamic vinegar
- ½ tsp. caraway seeds
- 2 tbsps. olive oil
- Black pepper
- 1 shredded red cabbage head

Directions:
1. In a bowl, combine the cabbage with the apples and the other ingredients, toss and serve.

Nutritional Information:
Calories: 165, Fat:7.4 g, Carbs:26 g, Protein:2.6 g, Sugars:2.6 g, Sodium:19 mg

Thyme Mushrooms

Prep time: 10 mins | Servings: 4

Ingredients:
- 1 tbsp. chopped thyme
- 2 tbsps. olive oil
- 2 tbsps. chopped parsley
- 4 minced garlic cloves
- Black pepper
- 2 lbs. halved white mushrooms

Directions:

1. In a baking pan, combine the mushrooms with the garlic and the other ingredients, toss, introduce in the oven and cook at 400 °F for 30 minutes.
2. Divide between plates and serve.

Nutritional Information:
Calories: 251, Fat:9.3 g, Carbs:13.2 g, Protein:6 g, Sugars:0.8 g, Sodium:37 mg

Rosemary Endives

Prep time: 10 mins | Servings: 4

Ingredients:
- 2 tbsps. olive oil
- 1 tsp. dried rosemary
- 2 halved endives
- ¼ tsp. black pepper
- ½ tsp. turmeric powder

Directions:

1. In a baking pan, combine the endives with the oil and the other ingredients, toss gently, introduce in the oven and bake at 400 °F for 20 minutes.
2. Divide between plates and serve.

Nutritional Information:
Calories: 66, Fat:7.1 g, Carbs:1.2 g, Protein:0.3 g, Sugars:1.3 g, Sodium:113 mg

Roasted Beets

Prep time: 10 mins | Servings: 4

Ingredients:
- 2 minced garlic cloves
- ¼ tsp. black pepper
- 4 peeled and sliced beets
- ¼ c. chopped walnuts
- 2 tbsps. olive oil
- ¼ c. chopped parsley

Directions:

1. In a baking dish, combine the beets with the oil and the other ingredients, toss to coat, introduce in the oven at 420 °F, and bake for 30 minutes.
2. Divide between plates and serve.

Nutritional Information:
Calories: 156, Fat:11.8 g, Carbs:11.5 g, Protein:3.8 g, Sugars:8 g, Sodium:670 mg

Minty Tomatoes and Corn

Prep time: 5 mins | Servings: 4

Ingredients:
- 2 c. corn
- 1 tbsp. rosemary vinegar
- 2 tbsps. chopped mint
- 1 lb. sliced tomatoes
- ¼ tsp. black pepper
- 2 tbsps. olive oil

Directions:

1. In a salad bowl, combine the tomatoes with the corn and the other ingredients, toss and serve.
2. Enjoy!

Nutritional Information:
Calories: 230, Fat:7.2 g, Carbs:11.6 g, Protein:4 g, Sugars:1 g, Sodium:53 mg

Pesto Green Beans

Prep time: 10 mins | Servings: 4

Ingredients:
- 2 tbsps. olive oil
- 2 tsps. sweet paprika
- Juice of 1 lemon
- 2 tbsps. basil pesto
- 1 lb. trimmed and halved green beans
- ¼ tsp. black pepper
- 1 sliced red onion

Directions:

1. Heat up a pan with the oil over medium-high heat, add the onion, stir and sauté for 5 minutes.
2. Add the beans and the rest of the ingredients, toss, cook over medium heat for 10 minutes, divide between plates and serve.

Nutritional Information:
Calories: 280, Fat:10 g, Carbs:13.9 g, Protein:4.7 g, Sugars:0.8 g, Sodium:138 mg

Sage Carrots

Prep time: 10 mins | Servings: 4

Ingredients:
- 2 tsps. sweet paprika
- 1 tbsp. chopped sage
- 2 tbsps. olive oil
- 1 lb. peeled and roughly cubed carrots
- ¼ tsp. black pepper
- 1 chopped red onion

Directions:

1. In a baking pan, combine the carrots with the oil and the other ingredients, toss and bake at 380 °F for 30 minutes.
2. Divide between plates and serve.

Nutritional Information:
Calories: 200, Fat:8.7 g, Carbs:7.9 g, Protein:4 g, Sugars:19 g, Sodium:268 mg

Dates and Cabbage Sauté

Prep time: 5 mins | Servings: 4

Ingredients:
- 2 tbsps. olive oil
- 2 tbsps. lemon juice
- 1 lb. shredded red cabbage
- Black pepper
- 8 pitted and sliced dates
- 2 tbsps. chopped chives
- ¼ c. low-sodium veggie stock

Directions:

1. Heat up a pan with the oil over medium heat, add the cabbage and the dates, toss and cook for 4 minutes.
2. Add the stock and the other ingredients, toss, cook over medium heat for 11 minutes more, divide between plates and serve.

Nutritional Information:
Calories: 280, Fat:8.1 g, Carbs:8.7 g, Protein:6.3 g, Sugars:4.7 g, Sodium:430 mg

Baked Squash Mix

Prep time: 10 mins | Servings: 4

Ingredients:
- 2 tsps. chopped cilantro
- 2 lbs. peeled and sliced butternut squash
- ¼ tsp. black pepper
- 1 tsp. garlic powder
- 2 tbsps. olive oil
- 1 tsp. chili powder
- 1 tbsp. lemon juice

Directions:

1. In a roasting pan, combine the squash with the oil and the other ingredients, toss gently, bake in the oven at 400 °F for 45 minutes, divide between plates and serve.

Nutritional Information:
Calories: 167, Fat:7.4 g, Carbs:27.5 g, Protein:2.5 g, Sugars:4.4 g, Sodium:10 mg

Kale Sauté

Prep time: 10 mins | Servings: 4

Ingredients:
- 1 chopped red onion
- 3 tbsps. coconut aminos
- 2 tbsps. olive oil
- 1 lb. torn kale
- 1 tbsp. chopped cilantro
- 1 tbsp. lime juice
- 2 minced garlic cloves

Directions:

1. Heat up a pan with the olive oil over medium heat, add the onion and the garlic and sauté for 5 minutes.
2. Add the kale and the other ingredients, toss, cook over medium heat for 10 minutes, divide between plates and serve.

Nutritional Information:
Calories: 200, Fat:7.1 g, Carbs:6.4 g, Protein:6 g, Sugars:1.6 g, Sodium:183 mg

Lemony Endives

Prep time: 10 mins | Servings: 4

Ingredients:
- 1 tbsps. grated lemon zest
- 4 halved endives
- 2 tbsps. olive oil
- 1 tbsp. lemon juice
- ¼ tsp. black pepper
- 2 tbsps. grated fat-free parmesan

Directions:

1. In a baking dish, combine the endives with the lemon juice and the other ingredients except the parmesan and toss.
2. Sprinkle the parmesan on top, bake the endives at 400 °F for 20 minutes, divide between plates and serve as a side dish.

Nutritional Information:
Calories: 71, Fat:7.1 g, Carbs:2.3 g, Protein:0.9 g, Sugars:2 g, Sodium:58 mg

Garlic Mushrooms and Corn

Prep time: 10 mins | Servings: 4

Ingredients:
- 2 c. corn
- 1 lb. halved white mushrooms
- ¼ tsp. black pepper
- ½ tsp. chili powder
- 2 tbsps. olive oil
- 1 c. no-salt-added, chopped and canned tomatoes
- 4 minced garlic cloves

Directions:

1. Heat up a pan with the oil over medium heat, add the mushrooms, garlic and the corn, stir and sauté for 10 minutes.
2. Add the rest of the ingredients, toss, cook over medium heat for 10 minutes more, divide between plates and serve.

Nutritional Information:
Calories: 285, Fat:13 g, Carbs:14.6 g, Protein:6.7 g, Sugars:2 g, Sodium:260 mg

Cilantro Broccoli

Prep time: 10 mins | Servings: 4

Ingredients:
- 2 tbsps. chili sauce
- 2 tbsps. olive oil
- 2 minced garlic cloves
- ¼ tsp. black pepper
- 1 lb. broccoli florets
- 2 tbsps. chopped cilantro
- 1 tbsp. lemon juice

Directions:

1. In a baking pan, combine the broccoli with the oil, garlic and the other ingredients, toss a bit, introduce in the oven and bake at 400 °F for 30 minutes.
2. Divide the mix between plates and serve.

Nutritional Information:
Calories: 103, Fat:7.4 g, Carbs:8.3 g, Protein:3.4 g, Sugars:33 g, Sodium:1.7 mg

Paprika Carrots

Prep time: 10 mins | Servings: 4

Ingredients:
- 1 tbsp. sweet paprika
- 1 tsp. lime juice
- 1 lb. trimmed baby carrots
- ¼ tsp. black pepper
- 3 tbsps. olive oil
- 1 tsp. sesame seeds

Directions:

1. Arrange the carrots on a lined baking sheet, add the paprika and the other ingredients except the sesame seeds, toss, introduce in the oven and bake at 400 °F for 30 minutes.
2. Divide the carrots between plates, sprinkle sesame seeds on top and serve.

Nutritional Information:
Calories: 142, Fat:11.3 g, Carbs:11.4 g, Protein:1.2 g, Sugars:7 g, Sodium:200 mg

Mashed Cauliflower

Prep time: 10 mins | Servings: 4

Ingredients:
- ½ c. coconut milk
- 1 tbsp. chopped chives
- 2 lbs. cauliflower florets
- ¼ tsp. black pepper
- 1 tbsp. chopped cilantro
- ½ c. low-fat sour cream

Directions:

1. Put the cauliflower in a pot, add water to cover, bring to a boil over medium heat, and cook for 25 minutes and drain.
2. Mash the cauliflower, add the milk, black pepper and the cream, whisk well, divide between plates, sprinkle the rest of the ingredients on top and serve.

Nutritional Information:
Calories: 188, Fat:13.4 g, Carbs:15 g, Protein:6.1 g, Sugars:5 g, Sodium:339 mg

Spinach Spread

Prep time: 10 mins | Servings: 4

Ingredients:
- 1 c. coconut cream
- 1 tbsp. chopped dill
- 1 lb. chopped spinach
- ¼ tsp. black pepper
- 1 c. shredded low-fat mozzarella

Directions:

1. In a baking pan, combine the spinach with the cream and the other ingredients, stir well, introduce in the oven and bake at 400 °F for 20 minutes.
2. Divide into bowls and serve.

Nutritional Information:
Calories: 340, Fat:33 g, Carbs:4 g, Protein:5 g, Sugars:3 g, Sodium:640 mg

Mustard Greens Sauté

Prep time: 10 mins | Servings: 4

Ingredients:
- 2 tbsps. olive oil
- 2 chopped spring onions
- 6 c. mustard greens
- 2 tbsps. sweet paprika
- Black pepper
- ½ c. coconut cream

Directions:
1. Heat up a pan with the oil over medium-high heat, add the onions, paprika and black pepper, stir and sauté for 3 minutes.
2. Add the mustard greens and the other ingredients, toss, cook for 9 minutes more, divide between plates and serve.

Nutritional Information:
Calories: 163, Fat:14.8 g, Carbs:8.3 g, Protein:3.6 g, Sugars:7 g, Sodium:390 mg

Basil Turnips Mix

Prep time: 10 mins | Servings: 4

Ingredients:
- ¼ c. low-sodium veggie stock
- 4 sliced turnips
- ¼ c. chopped basil
- 2 minced garlic cloves
- 1 tbsp. avocado oil
- ½ c. chopped walnuts
- Black pepper

Directions:
1. Heat up a pan with the oil over medium-high heat, add the garlic and the turnips and brown for 5 minutes.
2. Add the rest of the ingredients, toss, cook for 10 minutes more, divide between plates and serve.

Nutritional Information:
Calories: 140, Fat:9.7 g, Carbs:10.5 g, Protein:5 g, Sugars:3 g, Sodium:357 mg

Baked Mushrooms

Prep time: 10 mins | Servings: 4

Ingredients:
- Black pepper
- 1 tbsp. chopped chives
- 1 lb. small mushroom caps
- 1 tbsp. chopped rosemary
- 2 tbsps. olive oil

Directions:
1. Put the mushrooms in a roasting pan, add the oil and the rest of the ingredients, toss, bake at 400 °F for 25 minutes, divide into bowls and serve

Nutritional Information:
Calories: 215, Fat:12.3 g, Carbs:15.3 g, Protein:3.5 g, Sugars:4.5 g, Sodium:309 mg

Celery and Kale Mix

Prep time: 10 mins | Servings: 4

Ingredients:
- 5 c. torn kale
- 2 chopped celery stalks
- 1 tbsp. extra-virgin olive oil
- 3 tbsps. water

Directions:
1. Heat up a pan while using the oil over medium-high heat, add celery, stir and cook for 10 minutes.
2. Add kale and water, toss, cook for ten minutes more, divide between plates and serve.
3. Enjoy!

Nutritional Information:
Calories: 140, Fat:1 g, Carbs:6 g, Protein:6 g, Sugars:20 g, Sodium:169 mg

Spicy Avocado

Prep time: 10 mins | Servings: 1

Ingredients:
- 2 tbsps. hot sauce
- Sea salt
- 1 c. halved ripe avocado
- ½ Juiced lemon

Directions:
1. Slice the avocado in half a few times, spin and slice a few more times perpendicular to the first slices. You should end up with several cubes that are still attached to the peel.
2. Drizzle the lemon juice and hot sauce onto the avocado. Eat with a fork.

Nutritional Information:
Calories: 124, Fat:10.8 g, Carbs:9.5 g, Protein:1.9 g, Sugars:0.4 g, Sodium:95 mg

Cauliflower Risotto

Prep time: 10 mins | Servings: 4

Ingredients:
- 2 minced garlic cloves
- 1 tbsp. fresh lemon juice
- 2 tbsps. essential organic olive oil
- 2 tbsps. chopped thyme
- ¼ tsp. black pepper
- 12 oz. cauliflower rice
- Zest of ½ grated lemon

Directions:
1. Heat up a pan with the oil over medium-high heat, add cauliflower rice and garlic, stir and cook for 5 minutes.
2. Add freshly squeezed fresh lemon juice, lemon zest, thyme, salt and pepper, stir, cook for two main minutes more, divide between plates and serve.
3. Enjoy!

Nutritional Information:
Calories: 130, Fat:2 g, Carbs:6 g, Protein:8 g, Sugars:0.3 g, Sodium: 160 mg

Kale Dip

Prep time: 10 mins | Servings: 4

Ingredients:
- 1 c. coconut cream
- 1 tsp. chili powder
- 1 bunch kale leaves
- 1 chopped shallot
- ¼ tsp. black pepper
- 1 tbsp. olive oil

Directions:
1. Heat up a pan with the oil over medium heat, add the shallots, stir and sauté for 4 minutes.
2. Add the kale and the other ingredients, bring to a simmer and cook over medium heat for 16 minutes.
3. Blend using an immersion blender, divide into bowls and serve.

Nutritional Information:
Calories: 188, Fat:17.9 g, Carbs:7.6 g, Protein:2.5 g, Sugars:0.8 g, Sodium:23 mg

Dill Cabbage

Prep time: 10 mins | Servings: 4

Ingredients:
- 1 chopped yellow onion
- ¼ tsp. black pepper
- 1 lb. shredded green cabbage
- 1 tbsp. chopped dill
- 1 tbsp. olive oil
- 1 cubed tomato

Directions:
1. Heat up a pan with the oil over medium heat, add the onion and sauté for 5 minutes.
2. Add the cabbage and the rest of the ingredients, toss, cook over medium heat for 10 minutes, divide between plates and serve.

Nutritional Information:
Calories: 74, Fat:3.7 g, Carbs:10.2 g, Protein:2.1 g, Sugars:2 g, Sodium:115 mg

Curried Cauliflower Steaks with Red Rice

Prep time: 6 mins | Servings: 4

Ingredients:
- 1/3 c. extra-virgin olive oil
- 2 tsps. curry powder
- ½ tsps. kosher salt
- 2 cauliflower heads
- 1 tbsp. lemon juice
- 2 tbsps. chopped fresh cilantro
- 1 c. brown rice

Directions:
1. Preheat oven to 450 °F. Line a large baking sheet with tin foil.
2. Follow directions to prepare rice.
3. Whisk together oil, curry powder, and salt in a bowl.
4. Prepare cauliflower, making sure to keep stems intact. Place stem-side down on a cutting board and cut into thick slices to create "steaks." Get 4 steaks. Then slice the remaining cauliflower into smaller slices to get 4 cups.
5. Place steaks and florets onto a baking sheet. Brush both sides of the steaks with the curry mixture.
6. Place steaks in oven, turning after 15 minutes. Finish baking until steaks are tender and brown.
7. Divide rice evenly onto 4 plates and top each plate with a cauliflower steak. Sprinkle with cilantro.

Nutritional Information:
Calories: 410, Fat:21 g, Carbs:49 g, Protein:10 g, Sugars:5 g, Sodium:317 mg

Chapter 4 Poultry

Parmesan and Chicken Spaghetti Squash

Prep time: 5 mins | Servings: 6

Ingredients:
- 16 oz. mozzarella
- 1 spaghetti squash piece
- 1 lb. cooked cube chicken
- 1 c. Marinara sauce

Directions:
1. Split up the squash in halves and remove the seeds
2. Add 1 cup of water to the pot and place a trivet on top
3. Add the squash halves on the trivet
4. Lock up the lid and cook for 20 minutes at HIGH pressure
5. Do a quick release
6. Remove the squashes and shred them using a fork into spaghetti portions
7. Pour sauce over the squash and give it a nice mix
8. Top them up with the cubed up chicken and top with mozzarella
9. Broil for 1-2 minutes and broil until the cheese has melted

Nutritional Information:
Calories: 237, Fat:10 g, Carbs:32 g, Protein:11 g, Sugars:8 g, Sodium:900 mg

Apricot Chicken

Prep time: 25 mins | Servings: 4

Ingredients:
- 1 bottle creamy French dressing
- ¼ c. flavorless oil
- White cooked rice
- 1 large jar Apricot preserve
- 4 lbs. boneless and skinless chicken
- 1 package onion soup mix

Directions:
1. Rinse and pat dry the chicken. Dice into bite-size pieces.
2. In a large bowl, mix the apricot preserve, creamy dressing, and onion soup mix. Stir until fully combined.
3. Place the chicken in the bowl. Mix until coated.
4. In a large skillet, heat the oil. Place the chicken in the oil gently. Cook 4 – 6 minutes on each side, until golden brown.
5. Serve over rice.

Nutritional Information:
Calories: 202, Fat:12 g, Carbs:75 g, Protein:20 g, Sugars:10 g, Sodium:630 mg

Oven-fried Chicken Breasts

Prep time: 45 minutes | Servings: 8

Ingredients:
- ½ pack Ritz crackers
- 1 c. plain non-fat yogurt
- 8 boneless, skinless and halved chicken breasts

Directions:
1. Preheat the oven to 350 °F.
2. Rinse and pat dry the chicken breasts.
3. Pour the yogurt in a shallow bowl. Dip the chicken pieces in the yogurt, then roll in the cracker crumbs.
4. Place the chicken in a single layer in a baking dish.
5. Bake until golden brown on both sides, approximately 15 minutes per side.

Nutritional Information:
Calories: 200, Fat:13 g, Carbs:98 g, Protein:19 g, Sugars:1.5 g, Sodium:217 mg

Rosemary Roasted Chicken

Prep time: 10 mins | Servings: 8

Ingredients:
- 8 rosemary springs
- 1 minced garlic cloves
- Black pepper
- 1 tbsp. chopped rosemary
- 1 chicken
- 1 tbsp. organic olive oil

Directions:
1. In a bowl, mix garlic with rosemary, rub the chicken with black pepper, the oil and rosemary mix, place it inside roasting pan, introduce inside oven at 350 °F and roast for sixty minutes and 20 min.
2. Carve chicken, divide between plates and serve using a side dish.
3. Enjoy!

Nutritional Information:
Calories: 325, Fat:5 g, Carbs:15 g, Protein:14 g, Sugars:0 g, Sodium:1050 mg

Artichoke and Spinach Chicken

Prep time: 10 mins | Servings: 4

Ingredients:
- 10 oz. baby spinach
- ½ tsp. crushed red pepper flakes
- 14 oz. chopped artichoke hearts
- 28 oz. no-salt-added tomato sauce
- 2 tbsps. Essential olive oil
- 4 boneless and skinless chicken breasts

Directions:
1. Heat up a pan with the oil over medium-high heat, add chicken and red pepper flakes and cook for 5 minutes on them.
2. Add spinach, artichokes and tomato sauce, toss, cook for ten minutes more, divide between plates and serve.
3. Enjoy!

Nutritional Information:
Calories: 212, Fat:3 g, Carbs:16 g, Protein:20 g, Sugars:5 g, Sodium:418 mg

Pumpkin and Black Beans Chicken

Prep time: 10 mins | Servings: 4

Ingredients:
- 1 tbsp. essential olive oil
- 1 tbsps. Chopped cilantro
- 1 c. coconut milk
- 15 oz. drained and rinsed canned black beans
- 1 lb. skinless and boneless chicken breasts
- 2 c. water
- ½ c. pumpkin flesh

Directions:
1. Heat up a pan when using oil over medium-high heat, add the chicken and cook for 5 minutes.
2. Add the river, milk, pumpkin and black beans, toss, cover the pan, reduce heat to medium and cook for 20 mins.
3. Add cilantro, toss, divide between plates and serve.
4. Enjoy!

Nutritional Information:
Calories: 254, Fat:6 g, Carbs:16 g, Protein:22 g, Sugars:0.1 g, Sodium:92 mg

Chicken Thighs and Apples Mix

Prep time: 10 mins | Servings: 4

Ingredients:
- 3 cored and sliced apples
- 1 tbsp. apple cider vinegar treatment
- ¾ c. natural apple juice
- ¼ tsp. pepper and salt
- 1 tbsp. grated ginger
- 8 chicken thighs
- 3 tbsps. Chopped onion

Directions:
1. In a bowl, mix chicken with salt, pepper, vinegar, onion, ginger and apple juice, toss well, cover, keep within the fridge for ten minutes, transfer with a baking dish, and include apples.
2. Introduce inside oven at 400 °F for just one hour
3. Divide between plates and serve.
4. Enjoy!

Nutritional Information:
Calories: 214, Fat:3 g, Carbs:14 g, Protein:15 g, Sugars:10 g, Sodium:405 mg

Thai Chicken Thighs

Prep time: 10 mins | Servings: 6

Ingredients:
- ½ c. Thai chili sauce
- 1 chopped green onions bunch
- 4 lbs. chicken thighs

Directions:
1. Heat up a pan over medium-high heat.
2. Add chicken thighs, brown them for 5 minutes on both sides
3. Transfer to some baking dish then add chili sauce and green onions and toss.
4. Introduce within the oven and bake at 400°F for 60 minutes.
5. Divide everything between plates and serve.
6. Enjoy!

Nutritional Information:
Calories: 220, Fat:4 g, Carbs:12 g, Protein:10 g, Sugars:10 g, Sodium:1070 mg

Falling "Off" The Bone Chicken

Prep time: 10 mins | Servings: 4

Ingredients:
- 6 peeled garlic cloves
- 1 tbsp. organic extra virgin coconut oil
- 2 tbsps. Lemon juice
- 1 ½ c. pacific organic bone chicken broth
- ¼ tsp. freshly ground black pepper
- ½ tsp. sea flavored vinegar
- 1 whole organic chicken piece
- 1 tsp. paprika
- 1 tsp. dried thyme

Directions:
1. Take a small bowl and toss in the thyme, paprika, pepper and flavored vinegar and mix them. Use the mixture to season the chicken properly
2. Pour down the oil in your instant pot and heat it to shimmering, toss in the chicken with breast downward and let it cook for about 6-7 minutes
3. After the 7 minutes, flip over the chicken pour down the broth, garlic cloves and lemon juice
4. Lock up the lid and let it set for about 25 minutes on high setting.
5. Once done, let the cooker release its temperature naturally
6. Remove the dish from the cooker and let it stand for about 5 minute before serving.

Nutritional Information:
Calories: 664, Fat:44 g, Carbs:44 g, Protein:27 g, Sugars:0.1 g, Sodium:800 mg

Feisty Chicken Porridge

Prep time: 60 mins | Servings: 4

Ingredients:
- 1 ½ c. fresh ginger
- 1 lb. cooked chicken legs
- Green onions
- Toasted cashew nuts
- 5 c. chicken broth
- 1 cup jasmine rice
- 4 c. water

Directions:
1. Place the rice in your fridge and allow it to chill 1 hour prior to cooking
2. Take the rice out and add them to your Instant Pot
3. Pour broth and water
4. Lock up the lid and cook on Porridge mode
5. Release the pressure naturally over 10 minutes
6. Open the lid
7. Remove the meat from the chicken legs and add the meat to your soup
8. Stir well over sauté mode
9. Season with a bit of flavored vinegar and enjoy with a garnish of nuts and onion

Nutritional Information:
Calories: 206, Fat:8 g, Carbs:8 g, Protein:23 g, Sugars:0 g, Sodium:1050 mg

The Ultimate Faux-Tisserie Chicken

Prep time: 5 mins | Servings: 5

Ingredients:
- 1 c. low sodium broth
- 2 tbsps. Olive oil
- ½ quartered medium onion
- 2 tbsps. Favorite seasoning
- 2 ½ lbs. whole chicken
- Black pepper
- 5 large fresh garlic cloves

Directions:
1. Rub the chicken with 1 tablespoon of olive oil and sprinkle pepper on top
2. Place onion wedges and garlic cloves inside the chicken
3. Take a butcher's twin and secure the legs
4. Set your pot to Sauté mode
5. Add olive oil to a pan over medium heat, allow the oil to heat up
6. Add chicken and sear both sides for 4 minutes per side
7. Sprinkle your seasoning over the chicken, remove the chicken and place a trivet at the bottom of your pot
8. Sprinkle seasoning over chicken making sure to rub it
9. Transfer the chicken to the trivet with breast side facing up, lock up the lid
10. Cook on HIGH pressure for 25 minutes
11. Release the pressure naturally over 10 minutes
12. Allow it to rest and serve!

Nutritional Information:
Calories: 1010, Fat:64 g, Carbs:47 g, Protein:60 g, Sugars:1 g, Sodium:209 mg

Oregano Chicken Thighs

Prep time: 30 mins | Servings: 6

Ingredients:
- 12 chicken thighs
- 1 tsp. dried parsley
- ¼ tsp. pepper and salt.
- ½ c. extra virgin essential olive oil
- 4 minced garlic cloves
- 1 c. chopped oregano
- ¼ c. low-sodium veggie stock

Directions:
1. In your food processor, mix parsley with oregano, garlic, salt, pepper and stock and pulse.

2. Put chicken thighs within the bowl, add oregano paste, toss, cover and then leave aside within the fridge for 10 minutes.
3. Heat the kitchen grill over medium heat, add chicken pieces, close the lid and cook for twenty or so minutes with them.
4. Divide between plates and serve which has a side salad.
5. Enjoy!

Nutritional Information:
Calories: 254, Fat:3 g, Carbs:7 g, Protein:17 g, Sugars:0.9 g, Sodium:1030 mg

Pesto Chicken Breasts with Summer Squash

Prep time: 10 mins | Servings: 4

Ingredients:
- 4 medium boneless, skinless chicken breast halves
- 1 tbsp. olive oil
- 2 tbsps. Homemade pesto
- 2 c. finely chopped zucchini
- 2 tbsps. Finely shredded Asiago

Directions:
1. In a large nonstick skillet cook chicken in hot oil over medium heat for 4 minutes.
2. Turn chicken; add zucchini and/or squash. Cook for 4 to 6 minutes more or until the chicken is tender and no longer pink (170 °F) and squash is crisp-tender, stirring squash gently once or twice.
3. Transfer chicken and squash to 4 dinner plates. Spread pesto over chicken; sprinkle with Asiago

Nutritional Information:
Calories: 230, Fat:9 g, Carbs:8 g, Protein:30 g, Sugars:0.5 g, Sodium:578 mg

Chicken, Tomato and Green Beans

Prep time: 10 mins | Servings: 4

Ingredients:
- 6 oz. low-sodium canned tomato paste
- 2 tbsps. Olive oil
- ¼ tsp. black pepper
- 2 lbs. trimmed green beans
- 2 tbsps. Chopped parsley
- 1 ½ lbs. boneless, skinless and cubed chicken breasts
- 25 oz. no-salt-added canned tomato sauce

Directions:
1. Heat up a pan with 50 % with the oil over medium heat, add chicken, stir, cover, cook for 5 minutes on both sides and transfer to a bowl.
2. Heat inside the same pan while using rest through the oil over medium heat, add green beans, stir and cook for 10 minutes.
3. Return chicken for that pan, add black pepper, tomato sauce, tomato paste and parsley, stir, cover, cook for 10 minutes more, divide between plates and serve.
4. Enjoy!

Nutritional Information:
Calories: 190, Fat:4 g, Carbs:12 g, Protein:9 g, Sugars:8 g, Sodium:168 mg

Chicken Tortillas

Prep time: 10 mins | Servings: 4

Ingredients:
- 6 oz. boneless, skinless and cooked chicken breasts
- Black pepper
- 1/3 c. fat-free yogurt
- 4 heated up whole-wheat tortillas
- 2 chopped tomatoes

Directions:
1. Heat up a pan over medium heat, add one tortilla during those times, heat up and hang them on the working surface.

2. Spread yogurt on each tortilla, add chicken and tomatoes, roll, divide between plates and serve.
3. Enjoy!

Nutritional Information:
Calories:190 , Fat:2 g, Carbs:12 g, Protein:6 g, Sugars:2 g, Sodium:300 mg

---

Slow-roast Chicken with Homemade Gravy

Prep time: 15 mins | Servings: 6

Ingredients:
- 2 tbsps. Flour
- 1 tsp. Marmite
- 50g soft butter
- 1 lemon
- 2kg chicken
- 2 tsps. Fresh thyme leaves
- 1 lb. chicken stock

Directions:
1. Heat oven to 160C/140C fan/gas 3 and put the chicken in a roasting tin.
2. Put the butter into a small bowl and add the herbs and plenty of seasoning. Grate in the zest from the lemon and mash everything together with the butter using a fork. Rub this over the chicken breasts, legs and wings, then push the whole grated lemon into the big cavity of the chicken.
3. Pour half the stock into the tin. Use a large sheet of tin foil to cover the chicken and scrunch together the foil along the edges of the tin so the whole thing is sealed. Put in the oven and set your timer for 2 hrs.
4. Carefully remove the foil from the chicken, increase oven to 220C/200C fan/ gas 7 and put the chicken back in for another 30 minutes
5. After 30 minutes, take the chicken out of the oven and lift it onto a serving dish.
6. Snugly cover the chicken with foil and set aside while you make the gravy.
7. Tip the chicken juices and stock from the tin into a jug. Put the tin over a medium heat on your hob and use a wooden spoon to stir in the flour and Marmite, if using, with a splash of the juices to make a paste.
8. If you want, spoon the fat off the top of the chicken juices in the jug, then gradually stir this into the tin to make a smooth gravy.
9. Add as much of the rest of the stock as you need to make a good gravy, then serve with the chicken.

Nutritional Information:
Calories: 101.7, Fat:2.3 g, Carbs:8.3 g, Protein:11.3 g, Sugars:0.2 g, Sodium:433.3 mg

---

Balsamic Chicken Mix

Prep time: 10 mins | Servings: 4

Ingredients:
- 1 tsp. chopped rosemary
- 1 lb. chicken thighs
- 2 minced garlic cloves
- 1 grated orange zest
- 1/3 c. balsamic vinegar
- 1 tbsp. essential olive oil
- ½ c. cranberries
- 2 tsps. Chopped thyme

Directions:
1. Heat up a pan using the oil over medium-high heat, add chicken thighs skin side down, cook for 5 minutes and transfer to some plate.
2. Heat inside same pan over medium heat, add cranberries, garlic, vinegar, thyme, rosemary and orange zest, toss and bring to a simmer.
3. Return chicken to the pan as well, cook everything for ten mins, introduce the pan within the oven and bake at 325 ^{0}F for 25 minutes.
4. Divide between plates and serve.
5. Enjoy!

Nutritional Information:
Calories: 235, Fat:5 g, Carbs:14 g, Protein:15 g, Sugars:9 g, Sodium:185 mg

Turkey Pinwheels

Prep time: 5 mins | Servings: 4

Ingredients:
- 4 flour tortillas
- Grated carrots
- 2 deli-style turkey slices
- 2 Monterey Jack cheese slices
- 1 tbsp. Dijon mustard
- Romaine lettuce

Directions:
1. Spread mustard on each of the tortillas.
2. Top tortillas with cheese and turkey.
3. Add romaine lettuce and grated carrots. Roll up tightly. Cut each wrap into thirds.
4. Pack pinwheels with carrot sticks, grapes, a banana, or apple wedges.

Nutritional Information:
Calories: 206.9, Fat:8.9 g, Carbs:20.9 g, Protein:9.0 g, Sugars:0 g, Sodium:533.2 mg

Salsa Chicken

Prep time: 10 mins | Servings: 4

Ingredients:
- 1 ½ c. shredded fat-free cheddar cheese
- 16 oz. canned Salsa Verde
- ¼ c. chopped parsley
- Black pepper
- 1 merely lime juice
- 1 lb. skinless and boneless chicken breast
- 1 tbsp. organic essential olive oil

Directions:
1. Spread salsa inside a baking dish, add chicken at the very top, add oil, black pepper, lime juice, sprinkle cheese at the very top, introduce inside the oven at 400 °F and bake for one hour.
2. Sprinkle cilantro ahead, divide everything between plates and serve.
3. Enjoy!

Nutritional Information:
Calories: 250, Fat:1 g, Carbs:14 g, Protein:12 g, Sugars:4 g, Sodium:860 mg

Cajun Chicken and Rice

Prep time: 10 mins | Servings: 4

Ingredients:
- 1 tbsp. tomato sauce
- 1 tbsp. Cajun seasoning
- 1 ½ c. white rice
- 1 tbsp. olive oil
- 1 ¾ c. chicken broth
- 3 minced garlic cloves
- 1 lb. chicken breast
- 1 small diced onion
- 1 diced bell pepper

Directions:
1. Rinse the rice until the water runs clear
2. Cut the breast into half lengthwise and season both sides with the Cajun seasoning
3. Add rice, tomato paste, bell pepper and 1 teaspoon of Cajun seasoning and stir well
4. Pour broth over the rice and mix well
5. Arrange the chicken breast on top and lock up the lid, cook on High pressure for 7-8 minutes
6. Release the pressure naturally over 10 minutes
7. Shred the chicken with fork and stir well
8. Serve and enjoy with a drizzle of lime juice

Nutritional Information:
Calories: 210, Fat:8 g, Carbs:27 g, Protein:8 g, Sugars:0.5 g, Sodium:900 mg

Chicken, Scallions and Carrot Mix

Prep time: 10 mins | Servings: 6

Ingredients:
- 1 shredded small red cabbage head
- ¼ c. extra virgin olive oil
- Black pepper
- 1 c. grated carrot
- 4 c. cooked, boneless and shredded chicken
- 1/3 c. balsamic vinegar
- 6 sliced scallions

Directions:
1. In a bowl, mix extra virgin olive oil with vinegar and whisk.
2. In a salad bowl, mix chicken with scallions, cabbage, black pepper and carrot.
3. Add the vinegar and oil mix, toss and serve.
4. Enjoy!

Nutritional Information:
Calories: 170, Fat:2 g, Carbs:12 g, Protein:6 g, Sugars:2.3 g, Sodium:877 mg

Chicken and Bell Peppers

Prep time: 10 mins | Servings: 5

Ingredients:
- 4 chopped red sweet peppers
- 1 chopped yellow onion
- 1 c. shredded low-fat mozzarella cheese
- ¼ tsp. black pepper and salt
- 3 lbs. boneless and skinless chicken breasts
- 1 minced garlic herb
- 1 tbsp. coconut oil

Directions:
1. Put chicken in a baking dish greased using the oil, add garlic, peppers, salt and black pepper, cover with tin foil, introduce inside the oven and bake at 425 °F for 20 minutes.
2. Sprinkle the cheese, bake for ten minutes more, divide between plates and serve.
3. Enjoy!

Nutritional Information:
Calories: 225, Fat:12 g, Carbs:12 g, Protein:27 g, Sugars:4.8 g, Sodium:110 mg

Chicken Cranberry Meal

Prep time: 40-45 mins | Servings: 4-5

Ingredients:
- 1/3 c. balsamic vinegar
- 2 minced garlic cloves
- 1 grated orange zest
- 1 lb. bone-in chicken thighs
- 2 tsps. Chopped thyme
- 1 tbsp. olive oil
- ½ c. cranberries
- 1 tsp. chopped rosemary

Directions:
1. Preheat the oven to 325 °F.
2. Heat up the oil in a saucepan over medium-high flame; add the meat, skin side down and cook for 5 minutes.
3. Transfer to a plate and set aside.
4. In the same pan, add the cranberries, garlic, vinegar, thyme, rosemary, and orange zest; toss well and bring to a simmer.
5. Return the cooked chicken; stir and cook for 8-10 minutes.
6. Introduce in the oven and bake for 25 minutes
7. Serve warm!

Nutritional Information:
Calories: 257.1, Fat:2.8 g, Carbs:29.7 g, Protein:27.9 g, Sugars:26.4 g, Sodium:238.6 mg

Hot Chicken Mix

Prep time: 10 mins | Servings: 4

Ingredients:
- ½ c. hot sauce
- Black pepper
- 2 chopped green onions
- 1 c. coconut milk
- 1 ½ c. boneless and skinless chicken breasts
- A drizzle of organic olive oil
- 1 tsp. garlic powder

Directions:
1. Heat up a pan while using oil over medium-high heat
2. Add chicken, cook for 4 minutes on each side, add hot sauce, green onions, garlic powder, coconut milk and black pepper, toss, and cook for two minutes more.
3. Divide into bowls and serve.
4. Enjoy!

Nutritional Information:
Calories: 200, Fat:11 g, Carbs:14 g, Protein:11 g, Sugars:1 g, Sodium:4 mg

Asian Glazed Chicken

Prep time: 10 mins | Servings: 4

Ingredients:
- 3 tbsps. garlic
- ½ c. balsamic vinegar
- 3 tbsps. Garlic chili sauce
- ¼ c. olive oil
- 1/3 c. coconut aminos
- 1 tbsp. chopped green onion
- 8 de-boned and skinless chicken thighs
- ¼ tsp. black pepper

Directions:
1. Put the oil inside a baking dish, add chicken, aminos, vinegar, garlic, black pepper, onion and chili sauce, toss well, introduce inside oven and bake at 425 °F for thirty minutes.
2. Divide the chicken along with the sauce between plates and serve.
3. Enjoy!

Nutritional Information:
Calories: 254, Fat:12 g, Carbs:15 g, Protein: 20 g, Sugars:14.4 g, Sodium:1017 mg

Heavenly Garlic Chicken and Sprouts

Prep time: 10 mins | Servings: 4

Ingredients:
- 2 c. halved Brussels sprouts
- 1 tbsp. olive oil
- 30 whole garlic cloves
- 1 tbsps. Lemon juice
- 1 c. sliced yellow onion
- 1 ½ lbs. chicken pieces
- 1 fresh rosemary sprig

Directions:
1. Preheat the oven to 350°F.
2. In a skillet over medium, heat 1 tablespoon of olive oil.
3. Add the chicken, and brown each piece on each side.
4. Place the Brussels sprouts and onion in a large baking dish. Drizzle with the remaining olive oil and toss to coat.
5. Place the chicken over the vegetables and add the lemon juice, rosemary, and garlic.
6. Place in the oven and bake for approximately 1 hour, or until chicken is cooked through.

Nutritional Information:
Calories: 170.2, Fat:4.7 g, Carbs:19.5 g, Protein:12.9 g, Sugars:4 g, Sodium:400 mg

Italian Chicken Wings

Prep time: 10 mins | Servings: 4

Ingredients:
- 2 tbsps. Olive oil
- 1 tbsp. Italian seasoning
- 3 minced garlic cloves
- Black pepper
- 2 lbs. chicken wings
- 1 ¼ c. balsamic vinegar

Directions:
1. In a baking dish, mix chicken wings with Italian seasoning, garlic, vinegar, salt, pepper along while using extra virgin organic olive oil, toss to coat, introduce inside the oven at 425 °F and bake for an hour and fifteen minutes.
2. Divide everything between plates and serve.
3. Enjoy!

Nutritional Information:
Calories: 280, Fat:7 g, Carbs:12 g, Protein:14 g, Sugars:9.8 g, Sodium:454 mg

Smoked Chicken and Apple Mix

Prep time: ten mins | Servings: 6

Ingredients:
- ½ c. avocado mayonnaise
- 1 shredded carrot
- 1 chopped and cored red apple
- 1 tsp. chopped parsley
- ½ shredded small green cabbage head
- ½ c. de-boned, skinless and cooked smoked chicken
- 1 chopped celery rib

Directions:
1. In a bowl, mix chicken with celery, carrot, cabbage, apple, mayo and parsley, toss and serve cold.
2. Enjoy!

Nutritional Information:
Calories: 280, Fat:7 g, Carbs:10 g, Protein:13 g, Sugars:4 g, Sodium:500 mg

Creamy Chicken

Prep time: 15 mins | Servings: 6

Ingredients:
- Freshly ground black pepper
- 1 c. low-fat sour cream
- 1½ c. finely chopped fresh tomatoes
- 2 tbsps. Chopped fresh parsley
- 1 tsp. cayenne pepper
- 6 oz. skinless, de-boned chicken breasts
- ¾ c. low-fat, low-sodium chicken broth
- ½ tsp. ground cumin

Directions:
1. In a large slow cooker, add all ingredients except parsley and mix well.
2. Set the slow cooker on low.
3. Cover and cook for about 6 hours.
4. Serve this dish with the garnishing of chopped fresh parsley.

Nutritional Information:
Calories: 370.0, Fat:7.0 g, Carbs:54.0 g, Protein:22.0 g, Sugars:7 g, Sodium:890 mg

Chicken and Veggies

Prep time: 10 mins | Servings: 4

Ingredients:
- ½ c. chopped yellow onion
- 16 oz. cauliflower florets
- 2 tbsps. Organic olive oil
- ½ tsp. Italian seasoning
- 14 oz. chopped no-salt-added canned tomatoes
- 4 de-boned, skinless and cubed chicken breasts
- ¼ tsp. black pepper

Directions:
1. Heat up a pan while using the oil over medium-high heat, add chicken, black pepper, onion and Italian seasoning, toss and cook for 5 minutes.
2. Add tomatoes and cauliflower, toss, cover the pan and cook over medium heat for twenty possibly even minutes.
3. Toss again, divide everything between plates and serve.
4. Enjoy!

Nutritional Information:
Calories: 310, Fat:6 g, Carbs:14 g, Protein:20 g, Sugars:6 g, Sodium:550 mg

Hidden Valley Chicken Drummies

Prep time: 45 mins | Servings: 6 - 8

Ingredients:
- 2 tbsps. Hot sauce
- ½ c. melted butter
- Celery sticks
- 2 packages Hidden Valley dressing dry mix
- 3 tbsps. Vinegar
- 12 chicken drumsticks
- Paprika

Directions:
1. Preheat the oven to 350 ºF.
2. Rinse and pat dry the chicken.
3. In a bowl blend the dry dressing, melted butter, vinegar and hot sauce. Stir until combined.
4. Place the drumsticks in a large plastic baggie, pour the sauce over drumsticks. Massage the sauce until the drumsticks are coated.
5. Place the chicken in a single layer on a baking dish. Sprinkle with paprika.
6. Bake for 30 minutes, flipping halfway.
7. Serve with crudité or salad.

Nutritional Information:
Calories: 155, Fat:18 g, Carbs:96 g, Protein:15 g, Sugars:0.7 g, Sodium:340 mg

Lemon-parsley Chicken Breast

Prep time: 15 mins | Servings: 2

Ingredients:
- 1/3 c. lemon juice
- ¼ c. fresh parsley
- 1/3 c. white wine
- 3 tbsps. Bread crumbs
- 2 skinless and boneless chicken breasts
- 2 minced garlic cloves
- 2 tbsps. Flavorless oil

Directions:
1. Combine the wine, lemon juice and garlic in a measuring cup.
2. Pound each chicken breast, until they are ¼ inch thick.
3. Coat the chicken with bread crumbs, and heat the oil in a large skillet.
4. Fry the chicken for 6 minutes on each side, until they turn brown.
5. Stir in the wine mixture over the chicken.
6. Simmer for 5 minutes
7. Serve. Pour any extra juices over the chicken. Garnish with parsley.

Nutritional Information:
Calories: 117, Fat:12 g, Carbs:74 g, Protein:14 g, Sugars:5.8 g, Sodium:0 mg

Chicken and Brussels Sprouts

Prep time: 10 mins | Servings: 4

Ingredients:
- 1 cored, peeled and chopped apple
- 1 chopped yellow onion
- 1 tbsp. organic olive oil
- 3 c. shredded Brussels sprouts
- 1 lb. ground chicken meat
- Black pepper

Directions:
1. Heat up a pan while using oil over medium-high heat, add chicken, stir and brown for 5 minutes.
2. Add Brussels sprouts, onion, black pepper and apple, stir, cook for 10 minutes, divide into bowls and serve.
3. Enjoy!

Nutritional Information:
Calories: 200, Fat:8 g, Carbs:13 g, Protein:9 g, Sugars:3.3 g, Sodium:194 mg

Chicken Divan

Prep time: 45 minutes | Servings: 4

Ingredients:
- 1 c. croutons
- 1 c. cooked and diced broccoli pieces
- ½ c. water
- 1 c. grated extra sharp cheddar cheese
- ½ lb. de-boned and skinless cooked chicken pieces
- 1 can mushroom soup

Directions:
1. Preheat the oven to 350°F
2. In a large pot, heat the soup and water. Add the chicken, broccoli, and cheese. Combine thoroughly.
3. Pour into a greased baking dish.
4. Place the croutons over the mixture.
5. Bake for 30 minutes or until the casserole is bubbling and the croutons are golden brown.

Nutritional Information:
Calories: 380, Fat:22 g, Carbs:10 g, Protein:25 g, Sugars:2 g, Sodium:475 mg

Spicy Pulled Chicken Wraps

Prep time: 15 mins | Servings: 6-8

Ingredients:
- 1 head romaine lettuce
- 1½ tsps. Ground cumin
- 1½ c. low-fat, low-sodium chicken broth
- 1 tsp. paprika
- 1 tsp. garlic powder
- 1 lb. skinless, de-boned chicken breasts
- 2 tsps. Chili powder

Directions:
1. In a slow cooker add all ingredients except lettuce and gently, stir to combine.
2. Set the slow cooker on low.
3. Cover and cook for about 6-8 hours.
4. Uncover the slow cooker and transfer the breasts into a large plate.
5. With a fork, shred the breasts.
6. Serve the shredded beef over lettuce leaves.

Nutritional Information:
Calories: 150, Fat:3.4 g, Carbs:12 g, Protein:14 g, Sugars:7 g, Sodium:900 mg

Apricot Chicken Wings

Prep time: 15 mins | Servings: 3 - 4

Ingredients:
- 1 medium jar apricot preserve
- 1 package Lipton onion dry soup mix
- 1 medium bottle Russian dressing
- 2 lbs. chicken wings

Directions:
1. Pre-heat the oven to 350°F.
2. Rinse and pat dry the chicken wings.
3. Place the chicken wings on a baking pan, single layer.
4. Bake for 45 – 60 minutes, turning halfway.
5. In a medium bowl, combine the Lipton soup mix, apricot preserve and Russian dressing.
6. Once the wings are cooked, toss with the sauce, until the pieces are coated.
7. Serve immediately with a side dish.

Nutritional Information:
Calories: 162, Fat:17 g, Carbs:76 g, Protein:13 g, Sugars:24 g, Sodium:700 mg

Chicken and Broccoli

Prep time: 10 mins | Servings: 4

Ingredients:
- 2 minced garlic cloves
- 4 de-boned, skinless chicken breasts
- ½ c. coconut cream
- 1 tbsp. chopped oregano
- 2 c. broccoli florets
- 1 tbsp. organic olive oil
- 1 c. chopped red onions

Directions:
1. Heat up a pan while using the oil over medium-high heat, add chicken breasts and cook for 5 minutes on each side.
2. Add onions and garlic, stir and cook for 5 minutes more.
3. Add oregano, broccoli and cream, toss everything, cook for ten minutes more, divide between plates and serve.
4. Enjoy!

Nutritional Information:
Calories: 287, Fat:10 g, Carbs:14 g, Protein:19 g, Sugars:10 g, Sodium:1106 mg

Balsamic Roast Chicken

Prep time: 10 mins | Servings: 4

Ingredients:
- 1 tbsp. minced fresh rosemary
- 1 minced garlic clove
- Black pepper
- 1 tbsp. olive oil
- 1 tsp. brown sugar
- 6 rosemary sprigs
- 1 whole chicken
- ½ c. balsamic vinegar

Directions:
1. Combine garlic, minced rosemary, black pepper and the olive oil. Rub the chicken with the herbal olive oil mixture.
2. Put 3 rosemary sprigs into the chicken cavity.
3. Place the chicken into a roasting pan and roast at 400F for about 1 hr. 30 minutes.
4. When the chicken is golden and the juices run clear, transfer to a serving dish.
5. In a saucepan dissolve the sugar in balsamic vinegar over heat. Do not boil.
6. Carve the chicken and top with vinegar mixture.

Nutritional Information:
Calories: 587, Fat:37.8 g, Carbs:2.5 g, Protein:54.1 g, Sugars:0 g, Sodium:600 mg

Chicken, Bell Pepper & Spinach Frittata

Prep time: 15 mins | Servings: 8

Ingredients:
- ¾ c. frozen chopped spinach
- ¼ tsp. garlic powder
- ¼ c. chopped red onion
- 1 1/3 c. finely chopped cooked chicken
- 8 eggs
- Freshly ground black pepper
- 1½ c. chopped and seeded red bell pepper

Directions:
1. Grease a large slow cooker.
2. In a bowl, add eggs, garlic powder and black pepper and beat well.
3. Place remaining ingredients into prepared slow cooker.
4. Pour egg mixture over chicken mixture and gently, stir to combine.
5. Cover and cook for about 2-3 hours.

Nutritional Information:
Calories: 250.9, Fat:16.3 g, Carbs:10.8 g, Protein:16.2 g, Sugars:4 g, Sodium:486 mg

Hot Chicken Wings

Prep time: 25 mins | Servings: 4 - 5

Ingredients:
- 2 tbsps. Honey
- ½ stick margarine
- 2 tbsps. Cayenne pepper
- 1 bottle durkee hot sauce
- 10 - 20 chicken wings
- 10 shakes Tabasco sauce

Directions:
1. In a deep pot, heat the canola oil. Deep-fry the wings until cooked, approximately 20 minutes.
2. In a medium bowl, mix the hot sauce, honey, tabasco, and cayenne pepper. Mix well.
3. Place the cooked wings on paper towels. Drain the excess oil.
4. Toss the chicken wings in the sauce until coated evenly.

Nutritional Information:
Calories: 102, Fat:14 g, Carbs:55 g, Protein:23 g, Sugars:0.3 g, Sodium:340 mg

Balsamic Chicken and Beans

Prep time: 10 mins | Servings: 4

Ingredients:
- 1 lb. trimmed fresh green beans
- ¼ c. balsamic vinegar
- 2 sliced shallots
- 2 tbsps. Red pepper flakes
- 4 skinless, de-boned chicken breasts
- 2 minced garlic cloves
- 3 tbsps. Extra virgin olive oil

Directions:
1. Combine 2 tablespoons of the olive oil with the balsamic vinegar, garlic, and shallots. Pour it over the chicken breasts and refrigerate overnight.
2. The next day, preheat the oven to 375 °F.
3. Take the chicken out of the marinade and arrange in a shallow baking pan. Discard the rest of the marinade.
4. Bake in the oven for 40 minutes.
5. While the chicken is cooking, bring a large pot of water to a boil.
6. Place the green beans in the water and allow them to cook for five minutes and then drain.
7. Heat one tablespoon of olive oil in the pot and return the green beans after rinsing them.
8. Toss with red pepper flakes.

Nutritional Information:
Calories: 433, Fat:17.4 g, Carbs:12.9 g, Protein:56.1 g, Sugars:13 g, Sodium:292 mg

Butter Chicken

Prep time: 10 mins | Servings: 6

Ingredients:
- 8 finely chopped garlic cloves
- ¼ c. chopped low-fat unsalted butter
- Freshly ground black pepper
- 6 oz. skinless, de-boned chicken thighs
- 1 tsp. lemon pepper

Directions:
1. In a large slow cooker, place chicken thighs.
2. Top chicken thighs with butter evenly.
3. Sprinkle with garlic, lemon pepper and black pepper evenly.
4. Set the slow cooker on low.
5. Cover and cook for about 6 hours.

Nutritional Information:
Calories: 438, Fat:28 g, Carbs:14 g, Protein:30 g, Sugars:2 g, Sodium:700 mg

Five-Spice Roasted Duck Breasts

Prep time: 10 mins | Servings: 4

Ingredients:
- 1 tsp. five-spice powder
- ¼ tsp. cornstarch
- 2 orange juice and zest
- 1 tbsp. reduced-sodium soy sauce
- 2 lbs. de-boned duck breast
- ½ tsp. kosher salt
- 2 tsps. Honey

Directions:
1. Preheat oven to 375 °F.
2. Place duck skin-side down on a cutting board. Trim off all excess skin that hangs over the sides. Turn over and make three parallel, diagonal cuts in the skin of each breast, cutting through the fat but not into the meat. Sprinkle both sides with five-spice powder and salt.
3. Place the duck skin-side down in an ovenproof skillet over medium-low heat.
4. Cook until the fat is melted and the skin is golden brown, about 10 minutes. Transfer the duck to a plate; pour off all the fat from the pan. Return the duck to the pan skin-side up and transfer to the oven.
5. Roast the duck for 10 to 15 minutes for medium, depending on the size of the breast, until a thermometer inserted into the thickest part registers 150 °F.
6. Transfer to a cutting board; let rest for 5 minutes.
7. Pour off any fat remaining in the pan (take care, the handle will still be hot); place the pan over medium-high heat and add orange juice and honey. Bring to a simmer, stirring to scrape up any browned bits.
8. Add orange zest and soy sauce and continue to cook until the sauce is slightly reduced, about 1 minute. Stir cornstarch mixture then whisk into the sauce; cook, stirring, until slightly thickened, 1 minute.
9. Remove the duck skin and thinly slice the breast meat. Drizzle with the orange sauce.

Nutritional Information:
Calories: 152, Fat:2 g, Carbs:8 g, Protein:24 g, Sugars:5 g, Sodium:309 mg

Chicken and Radish Mix

Prep time: 10 minutes | Servings: 4

Ingredients:
- 10 halved radishes
- 1 tbsp. organic olive oil
- 2 tbsps. Chopped chives
- 1 c. low-sodium chicken stock
- 4 chicken things
- Black pepper

Directions:
1. Heat up a pan with all the oil over medium-high heat, add chicken, season with black pepper and brown for 6 minutes on either sides.

2. Add stock and radishes, reduce heat to medium and simmer for twenty minutes.
3. Add the chives, toss, divide between plates and serve.
4. Enjoy!

Nutritional Information:
Calories: 247, Fat:10 g, Carbs:12 g, Protein:22 g, Sugars:1.1 g, Sodium:673 mg

Chicken with Broccoli

Prep time: 15 mins | Servings: 4

Ingredients:
- 1 chopped small white onion
- 1½ c. low-fat, low-sodium chicken broth
- Freshly ground black pepper
- 2 c. chopped broccoli
- 1 lb. cubed, skinless and de-boned chicken thighs
- 2 minced garlic cloves

Directions:
1. In a slow cooker, add all ingredients and mix well.
2. Set slow cooker on low.
3. Cover and cook for 4-5 hours.
4. Serve hot.

Nutritional Information:
Calories: 300, Fat:9 g, Carbs:19 g, Protein:31 g, Sugars:6 g, Sodium:200 mg

Chicken, Pasta and Snow Peas

Prep time: 20 mins | Servings: 1 - 2

Ingredients:
- Fresh ground pepper
- 2 ½ c. penne pasta
- 1 standard jar tomato and basil pasta sauce
- 1 c. halved and trimmed snow peas
- 1 lb. chicken breasts
- 1 tsp. olive oil

Directions:
1. In a medium frying pan, heat the olive oil. Season the chicken breasts with salt and pepper. Cook the chicken breasts until cooked through for approximately 5 – 7 minutes each side.
2. Cook the pasta according to instructions on package. Cook the snow peas with the pasta.
3. Scoop 1 cup of the pasta water. Drain the pasta and peas, set aside.
4. Once the chicken is cooked, slice diagonally.
5. Add the chicken back to the frying pan. Add the pasta sauce. If the mixture seems dry.
6. Add some of the pasta water to desired consistency. Heat together.
7. Divide into bowls and serve immediately.

Nutritional Information:
Calories: 140, Fat:17 g, Carbs:52 g, Protein:34 g, Sugars:2.3 g, Sodium:400 mg

Chicken with Ginger Artichokes

Prep time: 10 mins | Servings: 4

Ingredients:
- 1 tbsp. grated ginger
- 2 tbsps. lemon juice
- ¼ tsp. black pepper
- 2 skinless, boneless and halved chicken breasts
- 1 c. no-salt-added and chopped canned tomatoes
- 2 tbsps. olive oil
- 10 oz. no-salt-added, drained and quartered canned artichokes

Directions:
1. Heat up a pan with the oil over medium heat, add the ginger and the artichokes, toss and cook for 5 minutes.
2. Add the chicken and cook for 5 minutes more.
3. Add the rest of the ingredients, bring to a simmer and cook for 20 minutes more.
4. Divide everything between plates and serve.

Nutritional Information:
Calories: 300, Fat:14.5 g, Carbs:16.4 g, Protein:15.1 g, Sugars:0 g, Sodium:377 mg

Roast Chicken Dal

Prep time: 10 mins | Servings: 4

Ingredients:
- 15 oz. rinsed lentils
- ¼ c. low-fat plain yogurt
- 1 minced small onion
- 4 c. de-boned, skinless and roasted chicken
- 2 tsps. Curry powder
- 1 ½ tsps. Canola oil
- 14 oz. fire-roasted diced tomatoes
- ¼ tsp. salt

Directions:
1. Heat oil in a large heavy saucepan over medium-high heat.
2. Add onion and cook, stirring, until softened but not browned, 3 to 4 minutes.
3. Add curry powder and cook, stirring, until combined with the onion and intensely aromatic, 20 to 30 seconds.
4. Stir in lentils, tomatoes, chicken and salt and cook, stirring often, until heated through.
5. Remove from the heat and stir in yogurt. Serve immediately.

Nutritional Information:
Calories: 307, Fat:6 g, Carbs:30 g, Protein:35 g, Sugars:0.1 g, Sodium:361 mg

Stovetop Barbecued Chicken Bites

Prep time: 10 minutes| Servings: 4

Ingredients:
- 1 diced medium bell pepper
- 1 tbsp. canola oil
- 1 c. tangy, spicy, and sweet barbecue sauce
- Freshly ground black pepper
- 1 diced medium onion
- 1 lb. de-boned skinless chicken breasts
- 3 minced garlic cloves

Directions:
1. Wash chicken breasts and pat dry. Cut into bite-sized chunks.
2. Heat oil in a large sauté pan over medium heat. Add chicken, onion, garlic, and bell pepper, and cook, stirring, for 5 minutes.
3. Add the barbecue sauce and stir to combine. Reduce heat to medium-low and cover pan. Cook, stirring frequently, until chicken is fully cooked, about 15 minutes.
4. Remove from heat. Season to taste with freshly ground black pepper and serve immediately.

Nutritional Information:
Calories: 191, Fat:5 g, Carbs:8 g, Protein:27 g, Sugars:0 g, Sodium:480 mg

Champion Chicken Pockets

Prep time: 5 mins | Servings: 4

Ingredients:
- ½ c. chopped broccoli
- 2 halved whole wheat pita bread rounds
- ¼ c. bottled reduced-fat ranch salad dressing
- ¼ c. chopped pecans or walnuts
- 1 ½ c. chopped cooked chicken
- ¼ c. plain low-fat yogurt
- ¼ c. shredded carrot

Directions:
1. In a small bowl stir together yogurt and ranch salad dressing.
2. In a medium bowl combine chicken, broccoli, carrot, and, if desired, nuts. Pour yogurt mixture over chicken; toss to coat.
3. Spoon chicken mixture into pita halves.

Nutritional Information:
Calories: 384, Fat:11.4 g, Carbs:7.4 g, Protein:59.3 g, Sugars:1.3 g, Sodium:368.7 mg

Peach Chicken Treat

Prep time: 30-35 mins | Servings: 4-5

Ingredients:
- 2 minced garlic cloves
- ¼ c. balsamic vinegar
- 4 sliced peaches
- 4 skinless, deboned chicken breasts
- ¼ c. chopped basil
- 1 tbsp. olive oil
- 1 chopped shallot
- ¼ tsp. black pepper

Directions:
1. Heat up the oil in a saucepan over medium-high flame.
2. Add the meat and season with black pepper; fry for 8 minutes on each side and set aside to rest in a plate.
3. In the same pan, add the shallot and garlic; stir and cook for 2 minutes.
4. Add the peaches; stir and cook for 4-5 more minutes.
5. Add the vinegar, cooked chicken, and basil; toss and simmer covered for 3-4 minutes more.
6. Serve warm.

Nutritional Information:
Calories: 270, Fat:0 g, Carbs:6.6 g, Protein:1.5 g, Sugars:24 g, Sodium:87 mg

Baked Chicken Pesto

Prep time: 10 mins | Servings: 4

Ingredients:
- 2 thinly sliced medium tomato
- 4 tsps. Basil pesto
- 6 tbsps. Shredded reduced fat mozzarella cheese
- 2 small de-boned, skinless chicken breast halves
- 4 tsps. grated parmesan cheese

Directions:
1. In cold water, wash chicken and dry using a paper towel. Create 4 thin slices out of chicken breasts by slicing horizontally.
2. At 400 °F, preheat oven then line a baking sheet with foil.
3. Put into the baking sheet the slices of chicken and spread at least 1 teaspoon of pesto on each chicken slice.
4. For 15 minutes, bake the chicken and ensure that the center is no longer pink. After which remove the baking sheet from the oven and top the chicken with parmesan cheese, mozzarella, and tomatoes.
5. Put into oven once again and heat for another 5 minutes to melt the cheese
6. Serve and enjoy.

Nutritional Information:
Calories: 163, Fat:5.9 g, Carbs:3.26 g, Protein:23.9 g, Sugars:1.8 g, Sodium:655 mg

Coconut-Crusted Lime Chicken

Prep time: 10 mins | Servings: 4

Ingredients:
- 50g desiccated coconut
- Mango chutney and rice
- 2 limes zest and juice
- 1 tsp. chilli powder
- 2 tsps. Medium curry powder
- 8 skinless, de-boned chicken thighs
- 1 tbsp. vegetable oil

Directions:
1. Heat oven to 200C/180C fan.
2. Put the chicken in a large bowl with the lime zest and juice, curry powder, chilli powder, if using, and seasoning.
3. Mix well, then toss in the coconut. Place chicken on a rack sitting in a roasting tin,

drizzle with the oil, then bake for 25 mins until cooked through and tender.
4. Serve with mango chutney, lime wedges for squeezing over and rice, if you like.

Nutritional Information:
Calories: 316, Fat:16 g, Carbs:2 g, Protein:41 g, Sugars:1 g, Sodium:600 mg

Chicken and Avocado Bake

Prep time: 10 mins | Servings: 4

Ingredients:
- 2 thinly sliced green onion stalks
- Mashed avocado
- 170 g non-fat Greek yogurt
- 1 ¼ g salt
- 4 chicken breasts
- 15 g blackened seasoning

Directions:
1. Start by putting your chicken breast in a plastic zip lock bag with the blackened seasoning. Close and shake, then marinate for about 2-5 minutes.
2. As your chicken is marinating, go ahead and put your Greek Yogurt, mashed avocado, and salt in your blender and pulse until smooth.
3. Place a large skillet or cast-iron pan on the stove at medium heat, oil the pan and cook the chicken until it is cooked through. You'll need about 5 minutes on each side. However, try not to dry the juices and plate it as soon as the meat is cooked.
4. Top with the yogurt mixture.

Nutritional Information:
Calories: 296, Fat:13.5 g, Carbs:6.6 g, Protein:35.37 g, Sugars:0.8 g, Sodium:173 mg

Balsamic Chicken over Greens

Prep time: 15 mins | Servings: 4

Ingredients:
- ¾ c. bottled balsamic vinaigrette salad dressing
- 8 oz. torn mixed greens
- 3 minced garlic cloves garlic
- 4 skinless, deboned chicken breast halves
- ¼ tsp. crushed red pepper

Directions:
1. Place chicken breast halves in a resealable plastic bag set in a shallow dish.
2. Stir together ½ cup of the vinaigrette, the garlic, and crushed red pepper. Pour marinade over the chicken.
3. Seal bag; turn to coat chicken. Marinate in the refrigerator for 1 to 4 hours, turning bag occasionally.
4. Drain chicken, reserving marinade. Place chicken on the rack of an uncovered grill directly over medium coals.
5. Grill for 12 to 15 minutes or until chicken is no longer pink (170 °F), turning once and brushing with the reserved marinade halfway through grilling time. Discard any remaining marinade.
6. Arrange greens on four dinner plates. Cut grilled chicken into strips. Arrange chicken on top of greens.
7. Serve with remaining ¼ cup vinaigrette

Nutritional Information:
Calories: 91.6, Fat:6.1 g, Carbs:3.2 g, Protein:6.6 g, Sugars:1 g, Sodium:312 mg

Chicken Chopstick

Prep time: 45 mins | Servings: 4

Ingredients:
- ¼ c. diced chopped onion
- 1 pack cooked chow Mein noodles
- Fresh ground pepper
- 2 cans cream mushroom soup
- 1 ¼ c. sliced celery
- 1 c. cashew nuts
- 2 c. cubed cooked chicken
- ½ c. water

Directions:
1. Preheat the oven to 375°F.

2. In a pot suitable for the oven, pour in both cans of cream of mushroom soup and water. Mix until combined.
3. Add the cooked cubed chicken, onion, celery, pepper, cashew nuts to the soup. Stir until combined. Add half the noodles to the mixture, stir until coated.
4. Top the casserole with the rest of the noodles.
5. Place the pot in the oven. Bake for 25 minutes.
6. Serve immediately.

Nutritional Information:
Calories: 201, Fat:17 g, Carbs:15 g, Protein:13 g, Sugars:7 g, Sodium:10 mg

Balsamic Turkey and Peach Mix

Prep time: 10 mins | Servings: 4

Ingredients:
- 4 sliced peaches
- ¼ tsp. black pepper
- 1 tbsp. avocado oil
- 1 skinless, boneless and sliced turkey breast
- 1 chopped yellow onion
- 2 tbsps. chopped chives
- ¼ c. balsamic vinegar

Directions:
1. Heat up a pan with the oil over medium-high heat, add the meat and the onion, toss and brown for 5 minutes.
2. Add the rest of the ingredients except the chives, toss gently and bake at 390 °F for 20 minutes.
3. Divide everything between plates and serve with the chives sprinkled on top.

Nutritional Information:
Calories: 123, Fat:1.6 g, Carbs:18.8 g, Protein:9.1 g, Sugars:6.6 g, Sodium:998 mg

Chicken and Asparagus Mix

Prep time: 10 mins | Servings: 4

Ingredients:
- ½ tsp. sweet paprika
- 2 chopped spring onions
- 2 tbsps. avocado oil
- 1 bunch trimmed and halved asparagus
- 14 oz. no-salt-added, drained and chopped canned tomatoes
- 2 skinless, boneless and cubed chicken breasts
- ¼ tsp. black pepper

Directions:
1. Heat up a pan with the oil over medium-high heat, add the meat and the spring onions, stir and cook for 5 minutes.
2. Add the asparagus and the other ingredients, toss, cover the pan and cook over medium heat for 20 minutes.
3. Divide everything between plates and serve.

Nutritional Information:
Calories: 171, Fat:6.4 g, Carbs:6.4 g, Protein:22.2 g, Sugars:0 g, Sodium:430 mg

Chicken and Dill Green Beans Mix

Prep time: 10 mins | Servings: 4

Ingredients:
- 10 oz. trimmed and halved green beans
- 1 chopped yellow onion
- ½ tsp. crushed red pepper flakes
- 2 tbsps. olive oil
- 1 tbsp. chopped dill
- 2 c. no-salt-added tomato sauce
- 2 skinless, boneless and halved chicken breasts

Directions:
1. Heat up a pan with the oil over medium-high heat, add the onion and the meat and brown it for 2 minutes on each side.
2. Add the green beans and the other ingredients, toss, introduce in the oven and bake at 380 °F for 20 minutes.
3. Divide between plates and serve right away.

Nutritional Information:
Calories: 391, Fat:17.8 g, Carbs:14.8 g, Protein:43.9 g, Sugars:1.7 g, Sodium:149 mg

Turkey with Beans and Olives

Prep time: 10 mins | Servings: 4

Ingredients:
- 1 lb. skinless, boneless and sliced turkey breast
- 1 c. pitted and halved green olives
- 1 c. no-salt-added tomato sauce
- 1 c. no-salt-added and drained black beans
- 1 tbsp. olive oil
- 1 tbsp. chopped cilantro

Directions:
1. Grease a baking dish with the oil, arrange the turkey slices inside, add the other ingredients as well, introduce in the oven and bake at 380 °F for 35 minutes.
2. Divide between plates and serve.

Nutritional Information:
Calories: 331, Fat:6.4 g, Carbs:38.5 g, Protein:30.7 g, Sugars:4.8 g, Sodium:616 mg

Parmesan Turkey

Prep time: 10 mins | Servings: 4

Ingredients:
- ½ c. grated low-fat parmesan
- 1 c. coconut milk
- 1 tbsp. olive oil
- 2 chopped shallots
- Black pepper
- 1 lb. skinless, boneless and cubed turkey breast

Directions:
1. Heat up a pan with the oil over medium-high heat, add the shallots, toss and cook for 5 minutes.
2. Add the meat, coconut milk, and black pepper, toss and cook over medium heat for 15 minutes more.
3. Add the parmesan, cook for 2-3 minutes, divide everything between plates and serve.

Nutritional Information:
Calories: 320, Fat:11.4 g, Carbs:14.3 g, Protein:11.3 g, Sugars:5 g, Sodium:990 mg

Chicken and Beets Mix

Prep time: 10 mins | Servings: 4

Ingredients:
- 2 peeled and shredded beets
- 1 c. skinless, deboned, cooked and shredded smoked chicken breast
- 1 shredded carrot
- 1 tsp. chopped chives
- ½ c. avocado mayonnaise

Directions:
1. In a bowl, combine the chicken with the beets and the other ingredients, toss and serve right away.

Nutritional Information:
Calories: 288, Fat:24.6 g, Carbs:6.5 g, Protein:14 g, Sugars:13 g, Sodium:504 mg

Turkey and Bok Choy

Prep time: 10 mins | Servings: 4

Ingredients:
- ½ c. low-sodium veggie stock
- 2 tbsps. olive oil
- 1 lb. torn bok choy
- 1 boneless, skinless and roughly cubed turkey breast
- 2 chopped scallions
- ¼ tsp. black pepper

- ½ tsp. grated ginger

Directions:
1. Heat up a pot with the oil over medium-high heat, add the scallions and the ginger and sauté for 2 minutes.
2. Add the meat and brown for 5 minutes more.
3. Add the rest of the ingredients, toss, simmer for 13 minutes more, divide between plates and serve.

Nutritional Information:
Calories: 125, Fat:8 g, Carbs:5.5 g, Protein:9.3 g, Sugars:2 g, Sodium:540 mg

Creamy Chicken and Shrimp Mix

Prep time: 10 mins | Servings: 4

Ingredients:
- 1 lb. skinless, boneless and cubed chicken breast
- 1 lb. peeled and deveined shrimp
- 1 tbsp. olive oil
- ¼ c. low-sodium chicken stock
- 1 tbsp. chopped cilantro
- ½ c. coconut cream

Directions:
1. Heat up a pan with the oil over medium heat, add the chicken, toss and cook for 8 minutes.
2. Add the shrimp and the other ingredients, toss, cook everything for 6 minutes more, divide into bowls and serve.

Nutritional Information:
Calories: 370, Fat:12.3 g, Carbs:12.6 g, Protein:8 g, Sugars:0.1 g, Sodium:274 mg

Allspice Chicken Wings

Prep time: 10 mins | Servings: 4

Ingredients:
- 2 tsps. ground allspice
- 2 tbsps. chopped chives
- Black pepper
- 2 lbs. chicken wings
- 2 tbsps. avocado oil
- 5 minced garlic cloves

Directions:
1. In a bowl, combine the chicken wings with the allspice and the other ingredients and toss well.
2. Arrange the chicken wings in a roasting pan and bake at 400 °F for 20 minutes.
3. Divide the chicken wings between plates and serve.

Nutritional Information:
Calories: 449, Fat:17 g, Carbs:1 g, Protein:6 g, Sugars:9 g, Sodium:113 mg

Cheddar Turkey Mix

Prep time: 10 mins | Servings: 4

Ingredients:
- 1 c. shredded fat-free cheddar cheese
- 1 lb. skinless, boneless and sliced turkey breast
- Black pepper
- 2 tbsps. chopped parsley
- 2 tbsps. olive oil
- 1 c. no-salt-added and chopped canned tomatoes

Directions:
1. Grease a baking dish with the oil, arrange the turkey slices into the pan, spread the tomatoes over them, season with black pepper, sprinkle the cheese and parsley on top, introduce in the oven at 400 °F and bake for 1 hour.
2. Divide everything between plates and serve.

Nutritional Information:
Calories: 350, Fat:13.1 g, Carbs:32.4 g, Protein:14 g, Sugars:12 g, Sodium:460 mg

Turkey with Celery Salad

Prep time: 4 mins | Servings: 4

Ingredients:
- 1 c. chopped celery stalks
- 1 c. pitted and halved black olives
- 2 c. skinless, boneless, cooked and shredded turkey breast
- 1 tbsp. olive oil
- 1 c. fat-free yogurt
- 2 chopped spring onions
- 1 tsps. lime juice

Directions:
1. In a bowl, combine the turkey with the celery and the other ingredients, toss and serve cold.

Nutritional Information:
Calories: 157, Fat:8 g, Carbs:10.8 g, Protein:11.5 g, Sugars:230 g, Sodium:0 mg

Lemony Leek and Chicken

Prep time: 10 mins | Servings: 4

Ingredients:
- 1 c. low-sodium veggie stock
- 4 roughly chopped leek
- ¼ tsp. black pepper
- 1 lb. skinless, boneless and cubed chicken breast
- 1 tbsp. no-salt-added tomato sauce
- ½ c. lemon juice
- 2 tbsps. avocado oil

Directions:
1. Heat up a pan with the oil over medium heat, add the leeks, toss and sauté for 10 minutes.
2. Add the chicken and the other ingredients, toss, cook over medium heat for 20 minutes more, divide between plates and serve.

Nutritional Information:
Calories: 1199, Fat:18.3 g, Carbs:16.6 g, Protein:26.5 g, Sugars:1 g, Sodium:50 mg

Chicken and Corn

Prep time: 10 mins | Servings: 4

Ingredients:
- 2 c. corn
- 1 c. low-sodium chicken stock
- 1 bunch chopped green onions
- 1 tsp. smoked paprika
- 2 tbsps. avocado oil
- ¼ tsp. black pepper
- 2 lbs. skinless, boneless and halved chicken breast

Directions:
1. Heat up a pan with the oil over medium-high heat, add the green onions, stir and sauté them for 5 minutes.
2. Add the chicken and brown it for 5 minutes more.
3. Add the corn and the other ingredients, toss, introduce the pan in the oven and cook at 390 ^{0}F for 25 minutes.
4. Divide the mix between plates and serve.

Nutritional Information:
Calories: 270, Fat:12.4 g, Carbs:12 g, Protein:9 g, Sugars:17 g, Sodium:586 mg

Chicken and Snow Peas

Prep time: 10 mins | Servings: 4

Ingredients:
- 1 chopped red onion
- 2 c. snow peas
- 2 tbsps. chopped parsley
- 2 lbs. skinless, boneless and cubed chicken breasts
- 2 tbsps. olive oil
- ¼ tsp. black pepper

- 1 c. no-salt-added canned tomato sauce

Directions:
1. Heat up a pan with the oil over medium heat, add the onion and the meat and brown for 5 minutes.
2. Add the peas and the rest of the ingredients, bring to a simmer and cook over medium heat for 25 minutes.
3. Divide the mix between plates and serve.

Nutritional Information:
Calories: 551, Fat:24.2 g, Carbs:11.7 g, Protein:69 g, Sugars:2 g, Sodium:681 mg

Turkey and Berries

Prep time: 10 mins | Servings: 4

Ingredients:
- 1 chopped red onion
- 1 c. low-sodium chicken stock
- ¼ c. chopped cilantro
- 2 lbs. skinless, boneless and cubed turkey breasts
- 1 c. cranberries
- Black pepper
- 1 tbsp. olive oil

Directions:
1. Heat up a pot with the oil over medium-high heat, add the onion, stir and sauté for 5 minutes.
2. Add the meat, berries and the other ingredients, bring to a simmer and cook over medium heat for 30 minutes more.
3. Divide the mix between plates and serve.

Nutritional Information:
Calories: 293, Fat:7.3 g, Carbs:14.7 g, Protein:39.3 g, Sugars:4 g, Sodium:595 mg

Balsamic Baked Turkey

Prep time: 10 mins | Servings: 4

Ingredients:
- 2 tbsps. balsamic vinegar
- 2 minced garlic cloves
- 1 skinless, boneless and sliced big turkey breast
- 1 tbsp. olive oil
- 1 tbsp. chopped cilantro
- Black pepper
- 1 tbsp. Italian seasoning

Directions:
1. In a baking dish, mix the turkey with the vinegar, the oil and the other ingredients, toss, introduce in the oven at 400 °F and bake for 40 minutes.
2. Divide everything between plates and serve with a side salad.

Nutritional Information:
Calories: 280, Fat:12.7 g, Carbs:22.1 g, Protein:14 g, Sugars:3 g, Sodium:760 mg

Turkey with Spiced Greens

Prep time: 10 mins | Servings: 4

Ingredients:
- Black pepper
- 1 c. mustard greens
- 1 tsp. ground allspice
- 1 lb. boneless, skinless and cubed turkey breast
- 1 tsp. ground nutmeg
- 1 tbsp. olive oil
- 1 chopped yellow onion

Directions:
1. Heat up a pan with the oil over medium-high heat, add the onion and the meat and brown for 5 minutes.
2. Add the rest of the ingredients, toss, cook over medium heat for 12 minutes more, divide between plates and serve.

Nutritional Information:
Calories: 270, Fat: 8.4g, Carbs:33.3 g, Protein:9 g, Sugars:0 g, Sodium:533 mg

Chapter 5 Fish and Seafood

Mighty Garlic and Butter Sword Fish

Prep time: 10 mins | Servings: 4

Ingredients:
- ½ c. melted butter
- 6 chopped garlic cloves
- 1 tbsp. black pepper
- 5 sword fish fillets

Directions:
1. Take a mixing bowl and toss in all of your garlic, black pepper alongside the melted butter
2. Take a parchment paper and place your fish fillet in that paper
3. Cover it up with the butter mixture and wrap up the fish
4. Repeat the process until all of your fish are wrapped up
5. Let it cook for 2 and a half hours and release the pressure naturally
6. Serve

Nutritional Information:
Calories: 379, Fat:26 g, Carbs:1 g, Protein:34 g, Sugars:0 g, Sodium:666 mg

Thai Coconut Tilapia and Rice

Prep time: 15 mins | Servings: 4

Ingredients:
- 170 g chopped baby spinach
- 425 g coconut milk
- 2 ½ g salted butter
- 680 g jasmine
- 2 ½ g chili flakes
- 4 coconut crusted tilapia fillets
- 680 g coconut water

Directions:
1. Preheat the oven to 400 °F and place fish in a lightly greased pan. Bake for 25 minutes.
2. In the meantime, put your rice in a pot to cook with coconut water, coconut milk, and a dash of salt. Set the pot at medium heat for about 2 minutes, till it reaches boiling point, then put the heat down and let the rice simmer for about twenty more minutes.
3. Add the chili flakes in now, to allow the rice to fully take in the flavor. Just before you are ready to serve, add in the spinach and stir for about 3 to 4 minutes, before straining both, and plating.
4. Take the fish out of the oven, slice, and serve over the coconut rice.

Nutritional Information:
Calories: 190, Fat:3.4 g, Carbs:35.67 g, Protein:6 g, Sugars:1.7 g, Sodium:256.2 mg

Supreme Cooked Lobster

Prep time: 10 mins | Servings: 4

Ingredients:
- 1 c. white wine
- 1 c. water
- 2 lobster pieces

Directions:
1. Add the listed ingredients to your Instant Pot
2. Lock up the lid and cook on HIGH pressure for 7 minutes
3. Release the pressure naturally
4. Open and add some extra melted butter
5. Serve and enjoy!

Nutritional Information:
Calories: 231, Fat:9 g, Carbs:5 g, Protein:30 g, Sugars:0 g, Sodium:551 mg

Tilapia with Parsley

Prep time: 10 mins | Servings: 6

Ingredients:
- 2 tbsps. Melted low-fat unsalted butter
- 1 tsp. garlic powder
- ¼ c. chopped fresh parsley
- Freshly ground black pepper
- 4 oz. tilapia fillets
- 3 tsps. Grated fresh lemon rind

Directions:
1. Grease a slow cooker.
2. Sprinkle the tilapia fillets with garlic powder and black pepper generously.
3. Place lemon rind and parsley over fillets evenly.
4. Drizzle with melted butter.
5. Set the slow cooker on low.
6. Cover and cook for about 1½ hours.

Nutritional Information:
Calories: 239.1, Fat:4.3 g, Carbs:22.3 g, Protein:33.7 g, Sugars:0 g, Sodium:381 mg

Pressure Cooker Crab Legs

Prep time: 5 mins | Servings: 4

Ingredients:
- 1 sliced lemon piece
- 1 c. water
- 1 c. melted butter
- 2 lbs. crab legs
- 1 c. white wine

Directions:
1. Add water to your Instant Pot alongside wine
2. Add crab legs
3. Lock up the lid and cook on HIGH pressure for 7 minutes
4. Release the pressure naturally over 10 minutes
5. Open the lid and add melted butter and a dash of lemon
6. Enjoy

Nutritional Information:
Calories: 191, Fat:1 g, Carbs:0 g, Protein:41 g, Sugars:0 g, Sodium:324 mg

Salmon and Broccoli Medley

Prep time: 1 min | Servings: 4

Ingredients:
- Crushed sunflower seeds
- 2 ½ oz. broccoli
- Fresh herbs
- 9 oz. new potatoes
- 2 ½ oz. salmon fillet
- 1 tsp. butter
- Pepper

Directions:
1. Chop the broccoli into florets and keep them on the side
2. Add ½ a cup of water to your Instant Pot
3. Season the potatoes with sunflower seeds, fresh herbs and pepper
4. Season the salmon and broccoli with sunflower seeds and pepper
5. Add potatoes to a steaming rack and smother them with butter
6. Transfer to your Instant Pot
7. Lock up the lid and cook for 2 minutes on the Steam setting
8. Quick release the pressure
9. Add broccoli florets and salmon and steam cook for 2 minutes more
10. Quick release
11. Serve and enjoy!

Nutritional Information:
Calories: 701, Fat:39 g, Carbs:30 g, Protein:57 g, Sugars:2 g, Sodium:190 mg

Tilapia with Lemon Garlic Sauce

Prep time: 5 mins | Servings: 4

Ingredients:
- 1 finely chopped garlic clove
- 1 tbsp. olive oil
- Pepper
- 3 tbsps. Fresh lemon juice
- 4 tilapia fillets
- 1 tsp. dried parsley flakes

Directions:
1. First, spray baking dish with non-stick cooking spray then preheat oven at 375 °F.
2. In cool water, rinse tilapia fillets and using paper towels pat dry.
3. Place tilapia fillets in the baking dish then pour olive oil and lemon juice and top off with pepper, parsley and garlic.
4. Bake tilapia in the preheated oven for 15 minutes.
5. Remove from oven and let it rest for 5 minutes.
6. Enjoy!

Nutritional Information:
Calories: 155, Fat:5.7 g, Carbs:2.1 g, Protein:23.7 g, Sugars:0.5 g, Sodium:116.7 mg

Easy Coconut Shrimp

Prep time: 5 mins | Servings: 2

Ingredients:
- 12 deveined and peeled large shrimp
- ¼ c. panko breadcrumbs
- ½ tsp. kosher salt
- ¼ c. sweetened coconut
- ½ c. coconut milk

Directions:
1. Heat the oven to 375 F.
2. Coat a baking sheet lightly with cooking spray.
3. Put the coconut, panko and salt in a food processor and pulse.
4. In a small bowl pour in the coconut milk.
5. Dip each shrimp first into the coconut milk and then into the panko mixture. Place on to the greased baking sheet.
6. Lightly spray the tops of the shrimp with cooking spray.
7. Bake about 10 to 15 minutes until golden brown.

Nutritional Information:
Calories: 300.2, Fat:13.4 g, Carbs:17.2 g, Protein:27.5 g, Sugars:1.7 g, Sodium:588.7 mg

Shrimp Quesadillas

Prep time: 16 mins | Servings: 1 - 2

Ingredients:
- Two whole wheat tortillas
- ½ tsp. ground cumin
- 4 cilantro leaves
- 3 oz. diced cooked shrimp
- 1 de-seeded plump tomato
- ¾ c. grated non-fat mozzarella cheese
- ¼ c. diced red onion

Directions:
1. In medium bowl, combine the grated mozzarella cheese and the warm, cooked shrimp. Add the ground cumin, red onion, and tomato. Mix together. Spread the mixture evenly on the tortillas.
2. Heat a non-stick frying pan. Place the tortillas in the pan, then heat until they crisp.
3. Add the cilantro leaves. Fold over the tortillas.
4. Press down for 1 – 2 minutes. Slice the tortillas into wedges.
5. Serve immediately.

Nutritional Information:
Calories: 99, Fat:9 g, Carbs:7.2 g, Protein:59 g, Sugars:4 g, Sodium:500 mg

The OG Tuna Sandwich

Prep time: 15 mins | Servings: 2

Ingredients:
- 30 g olive oil
- 1 peeled and diced medium cucumber
- 2 ½ g pepper
- 4 whole wheat bread slices
- 85 g diced onion
- 2 ½ g salt
- 1 can flavored tuna
- 85 g shredded spinach

Directions:
1. Grab your blender and add the spinach, tuna, onion, oil, salt and pepper in, and pulse for about 10 to 20 seconds.
2. In the meantime, toast your bread and add your diced cucumber to a bowl, which you can pour your tuna mixture in. Carefully mix and add the mixture to the bread once toasted.
3. Slice in half and serve, while storing the remaining mixture in the fridge.

Nutritional Information:
Calories: 302, Fat:5.8 g, Carbs:36.62 g, Protein:28 g, Sugars:3.22 g, Sodium:445 mg

Easy To Understand Mussels

Prep time: 10 mins | Servings: 4

Ingredients:
- 2 lbs. cleaned mussels
- 4 minced garlic cloves
- 2 chopped shallots
- Lemon and parsley
- 2 tbsps. Butter
- ½ c. broth
- ½ c. white wine

Directions:
1. Clean the mussels and remove the beard
2. Discard any mussels that do not close when tapped against a hard surface
3. Set your pot to Sauté mode and add chopped onion and butter
4. Stir and sauté onions
5. Add garlic and cook for 1 minute
6. Add broth and wine
7. Lock up the lid and cook for 5 minutes on HIGH pressure
8. Release the pressure naturally over 10 minutes
9. Serve with a sprinkle of parsley and enjoy!

Nutritional Information:
Calories: 286, Fat:14 g, Carbs:12 g, Protein:28 g, Sugars:0 g, Sodium:314 mg

Chili-Rubbed Tilapia with Asparagus & Lemon

Prep time: 1o mins | Servings: 4

Ingredients:
- 3 tbsps. Lemon juice
- 2 tbsps. Chili powder
- 2 tbsps. Extra-virgin olive oil
- ½ tsp. divided salt
- 2 lbs. trimmed asparagus
- ½ tsp. garlic powder
- 1 lb. tilapia fillets

Directions:
1. Bring 1 inch of water to a boil in a large saucepan. Put asparagus in a steamer basket, place in the pan, cover and steam until tender-crisp, about 4 minutes.
2. Transfer to a large plate, spreading out to cool.
3. Combine chili powder, garlic powder and ¼ teaspoon salt on a plate. Dredge fillets in the spice mixture to coat. Heat oil in a large nonstick skillet over medium-high heat. Add the fish and cook until just opaque in the center, gently turning halfway, and 5 to 7 minutes total.

4. Divide among 4 plates. Immediately add lemon juice, the remaining ¼ teaspoon salt and asparagus to the pan and cook, stirring constantly, until the asparagus is coated and heated through, about 2 minutes.
5. Serve the asparagus with the fish.

Nutritional Information:
Calories: 211, Fat:10 g, Carbs:8 g, Protein:26 g, Sugars:0.4 g, Sodium:375.7 mg

Parmesan-Crusted Fish

Prep time: 5 mins | Servings: 4

Ingredients:
- ¾ tsp. ground ginger
- 1/3 c. panko bread crumbs
- Mixed fresh salad greens
- ¼ c. finely shredded parmesan cheese
- 1 tbsp. butter
- 4 skinless cod fillets
- 3 c. julienned carrots

Directions:
1. Preheat oven to 450 °F. Lightly coat a baking sheet with nonstick cooking spray.
2. Rinse and pat dry fish; place on baking sheet. Season with salt and pepper.
3. In small bowl stir together crumbs and cheese; sprinkle on fish.
4. Bake, uncovered, 4 to 6 minutes for each 1/2-inch thickness of fish, until crumbs are golden and fish flakes easily when tested with a fork.
5. Meanwhile, in a large skillet bring 1/2 cup water to boiling; add carrots. Reduce heat.
6. Cook, covered, for 5 minutes. Uncover; cook 2 minutes more. Add butter and ginger; toss.
7. Serve fish and carrots with greens.

Nutritional Information:
Calories: 216.4, Fat:10.1 g, Carbs:1.3 g, Protein:29.0 g, Sugars:0.1 g, Sodium:428.3 mg

Tuna Melt Delight

Prep time: 10 mins | Servings: 2

Ingredients:
- 3 oz. grated reduced-fat cheddar cheese
- 1/3 c. chopped celery
- Pepper and salt
- ¼ c. chopped onion
- 2 whole-wheat English muffins
- 6 oz. drained white tuna
- ¼ c. low fat Thousand Island salad dressing

Directions:
1. Preheat broiler.
2. Mix together tuna, celery, onion and salad dressing.
3. Season with salt and pepper.
4. Toast English muffin halves.
5. Place split-side-up on baking sheet and top each muffin with 1/4 of tuna mixture.
6. Broil 2-3 minutes or until heated through.
7. Top with cheese and return to broiler until cheese is melted and bubbly, about 1 minute.

Nutritional Information:
Calories: 186.2, Fat:7.7 g, Carbs:18.0 g, Protein:11.7 g, Sugars:0.3 g, Sodium:534.9 mg

Uber-Cool Salmon Steaks

Prep time: 5 mins | Servings: 4-6

Ingredients:
- 2 lbs. salmon steaks
- Crushed sunflower seeds
- 1/8 tsp. black pepper
- ½ c. water
- 1 sliced medium-sized onion
- ½ c. dry white wine
- 1 sliced lemon

Directions:

1. Place a trivet in your cooker
2. Add water and wine and sprinkle sunflower seeds and pepper
3. Arrange the lemon slices over fish
4. Make sure to reserve 4 slices for garnish
5. Lock up the lid and cook on HIGH pressure for 6 minutes
6. Release the pressure naturally over 10 minutes
7. Place the fish on serving dish
8. Discard the onion and lemon
9. Serve with garnish and reserved lemon slices
10. Enjoy!

Nutritional Information:
Calories: 558, Fat:36 g, Carbs:10 g, Protein:49 g, Sugars:0 g, Sodium:107 mg

Crustless Crab "Quiche"

Prep time: 10 mins | Servings: 5

Ingredients:
- 8 oz. crab meat
- 1 c. half and half
- 1 tsp. sweet smoked paprika
- 1 c. chopped green onion
- 1 tsp. Herbes de Provence
- 4 whole eggs
- 1 tsp. pepper
- 1 c. shredded parmesan

Directions:
1. Take a large sized bowl and add eggs, half and half and whisk
2. Add pepper, sweet smoked paprika, Herbes De Provence and shredded cheese, stir well
3. Stir in chopped green onion
4. Add crab meat and mix well
5. Lay out aluminum foil bigger than your pan
6. Place a spring form pan on the sheet and crimp the sheet about the bottom
7. Add egg mixture to the pan
8. Cover loosely with foil
9. Add 2 cups of water to the pot
10. Place a steamer rack in the pot
11. Place the spring form pan on the trivet
12. Lock up the lid and cook on HIGH pressure for 40 minutes
13. Release the pressure naturally over 10 minutes
14. Take the hot silicone pan out and loosen the edges of the quiche
15. Remove the outer ring and serve the quiche
16. Enjoy!

Nutritional Information:
Calories: 602, Fat:44 g, Carbs:18 g, Protein:33 g, Sugars:2.4 g, Sodium:940.6 mg

Godly Garlic Butter Salmon Asparagus

Prep time: 5 mins | Servings: 4

Ingredients:
- Red pepper flakes
- 1 lb. asparagus
- 1 ½ tbsps. Minced garlic
- ¼ c. lemon juice
- Honey
- 1 lb. sliced salmon fillet
- 3 tbsps. Butter

Directions:
1. Take 3 large pieces of oil and lay them on a flat surface
2. Curve the edge so lemon juice does not fall and divide asparagus equally amongst the packets
3. Slater each piece with ½ a tablespoon of garlic and place them on top of the asparagus
4. Add 1 tablespoon of lemon juice over the salmon
5. Sprinkle red pepper flakes and drizzle honey
6. Add 1 tablespoon of butter on top of each salmon
7. Seal the foil properly
8. Add 1 and a ½ a cup of water to the pot
9. Place a metal trivet to the pot

10. Place 3 foil packets on top of the trivet
11. Lock up the lid and cook on STEAM setting for 4 minutes
12. Quick release the pressure
13. Use tongs to take the foil out
14. Transfer the contents of the pack to a plate alongside the juices
15. Enjoy!

Nutritional Information:
Calories: 909, Fat:60 g, Carbs:6 g, Protein:83 g, Sugars:2 g, Sodium:970 mg

---

Steamed Blue Crabs

Prep time: 30 mins | Servings: 6

Ingredients:
- 3 c. distilled white vinegar
- 3 c. beer
- 30 live blue crabs
- ¼ c. salt
- ½ c. seafood seasoning

Directions:
1. In a large stock pot, combine the seasoning, salt, beer and white vinegar. Bring it to a boil.
2. Place each crab upside down and stick a knife into the shell, just before cooking them. Cover the lid, leaving a crack for the steam to vent.
3. Steam the crabs until they turn bright orange, and float to the top. Allow them to cook for another 2 - 3 minutes.
4. Serve immediately.

Nutritional Information:
Calories: 77, Fat:7 g, Carbs:31 g, Protein:9.8 g, Sugars:0 g, Sodium:237 mg

---

Capelin Balls

Prep time: 20 mins | Servings: 4

Ingredients:
- 2 beaten egg whites
- ½ c. milk
- 8 oz. de-boned capelin fish head
- 2 tbsps. Rice

Directions:
1. Rinse the rice and place into 2 oz. boiling water. Cook on low heat until done.
2. Mix the fish meat with the cooked rice, add egg whites and milk and stir.
3. Form the balls and cook in a steamer for 30 min or until soft.
4. Serve with sour cream.

Nutritional Information:
Calories: 230, Fat:5.7 g, Carbs:22 g, Protein:19.3 g, Sugars:0 g, Sodium:173.1 mg

---

Southwestern Salmon

Prep time: 5 minutes | Servings 4

Ingredients:
- 1 lb. de-boned salmon fillet
- 1 tsp. ground cumin
- 1/8 tsp. ground cayenne pepper
- 1 tsp. ground paprika
- ½ tsp. ground coriander
- 1 tsp. dried cilantro
- ½ tsp. freshly ground black pepper

Directions:
1. Move a rack to the top of the oven and preheat broiler. Spray a baking sheet lightly with oil and set aside.
2. Place the seasonings into a small bowl and mix well to combine.
3. Sprinkle the spice mixture over the salmon fillet and gently rub the mixture into the fish. Place the fillet on the prepared baking sheet.
4. Place the sheet on the top rack in the oven and broil for about 7 minutes; 1–2 minutes less for thin fillets, a little longer for thicker

fillets. When cooked fully, salmon will be opaque and flake easily.
5. Remove sheet from oven, slice salmon into 4 portions, and serve immediately.

Nutritional Information:
Calories: 171, Fat:8 g, Carbs:0 g, Protein:22 g, Sugars:3 g, Sodium:380.8 mg

Pressure Cooker Salmon Steaks

Prep time: 5 mins | Servings: 2-3

Ingredients:
- 1 thinly sliced medium onion
- 1 thinly sliced lemon
- 1 tsp. black pepper
- 3 lbs. salmon steaks
- 1 ½ c. water

Directions:
1. Prepare your pressure cooker by placing a trivet inside. Pour in the water.
2. Season the fish with the pepper and place it on the trivet.
3. Arrange the lemon and onion slices on top of the fish but reserve a few lemon slices for garnish.
4. Close and lock the lid. Cook on high pressure for 6 minutes. When the cooking time is up, release the pressure using the quick release method.
5. Open the cooker, remove the fish and place it on a serving dish.
6. Discard the lemon and onion slices. Garnish the fish with a few lemon slices and serve hot.

Nutritional Information:
Calories: 264, Fat:7 g, Carbs:4 g, Protein:10 g, Sugars:0 g, Sodium:138 mg

Salmon and Horseradish Sauce

Prep time: 10 mins | Servings: 4

Ingredients:
- ½ c. coconut cream
- 1 tbsps. Prepared horseradish
- 4 de-boned medium salmon fillets
- 2 tbsps. Chopped dill
- 1 ½ tbsps. Organic olive oil
- ¼ tsp. black pepper

Directions:
1. Heat up a pan while using the oil over medium-high heat, add salmon fillets, season with black pepper and cook for 5 minutes one each side.
2. In a bowl, combine the cream with the dill and horseradish and whisk well.
3. Divide the salmon between plates and serve with all the horseradish cream for the top.
4. Enjoy!

Nutritional Information:
Calories: 275, Fat:12 g, Carbs:14 g, Protein:27 g, Sugars:1 g, Sodium:801.8 mg

Simple Grilled Tilapia

Prep time: 10 mins | Servings: 4

Ingredients:
- 4 medium tilapia fillets
- 1 tsp. smoked paprika
- ¼ tsp. black pepper
- 1 ½ tbsps. Extra virgin extra virgin olive oil
- ½ tsp. garlic powder

Directions:
1. Heat up a pan while using oil over medium-high heat, season the fish with paprika, garlic powder and black pepper, add it for the pan, cook for 4 minutes on them, divide between plates and serve employing a side salad.
2. Enjoy!

Nutritional Information:
Calories: 222, Fat:4 g, Carbs:14 g, Protein:25 g, Sugars:1 g, Sodium:250 mg

Crunchy Topped Fish with Potato Sticks

Prep time: 5 mins | Servings: 4

Ingredients:
- 2 tbsps. Melted margarine
- Nonstick spray coating
- ¾ c. crushed herb-seasoned stuffing mix
- 12 oz. sliced medium baking potatoes
- 2 tsps. Melted cooking oil
- 16 oz. fresh catfish fillets
- Garlic salt

Directions:
1. Rinse fish and pat dry with paper towels; set aside.
2. Line a large baking sheet with foil. Spray foil with nonstick spray coating.
3. Arrange potato sticks in a single layer over half of the baking sheet. Brush potatoes with oil or the 2 teaspoons melted margarine. Sprinkle with garlic salt.
4. Bake in a 450 degree F oven for 10 minutes.
5. Meanwhile, stir together stuffing mix and the 2 tablespoons melted margarine.
6. Place fish on baking sheet next to potatoes. Sprinkle stuffing mix over fish. Return pan to oven and bake 9 to 12 minutes more or until fish flakes easily when tested with a fork and potatoes are tender.

Nutritional Information:
Calories: 94, Fat: 6.19g, Carbs:9.6 g, Protein:1.2 g, Sugars:1 g, Sodium:630 mg

Easy Sautéed Fish Fillets

Prep time: 5 mins | Servings: 4

Ingredients:
- 1 tbsp. extra-virgin olive oil
- ½ tsp. salt
- 1 lb. sliced haddock
- 1/3 c. all-purpose flour
- Freshly ground pepper

Directions:
1. Combine flour, salt and pepper in a shallow dish; thoroughly dredge fillets
2. Heat oil in a large nonstick skillet over medium-high heat.
3. Add the fish, working in batches if necessary, and cook until lightly browned and just opaque in the center, 3 to 4 minutes per side.
4. Serve immediately.

Nutritional Information:
Calories: 111, Fat:11 g, Carbs:15 g, Protein:13 g, Sugars:0 g, Sodium:481.4 mg

Tasty Halibut and Cherry Tomatoes

Prep time: 10 mins | Servings: 4

Ingredients:
- 3 minced garlic cloves
- 4 skinless halibut fillets
- 2 c. cherry tomatoes
- 2 tbsps. Chopped basil
- ¼ tsp. black pepper
- 1 ½ tbsps. Organic olive oil
- 2 tbsps. Balsamic vinegar

Directions:
1. Heat up a pan with 1 tablespoon organic essential olive oil, add halibut fillets, cook them for 5 minutes on both sides and divide between plates.
2. Heat up another pan because of the rest within the oil over medium-high heat, add the tomatoes, garlic, vinegar and basil, toss, cook for 3 minutes, add next on the fish and serve.
3. Enjoy!

Nutritional Information:
Calories: 221, Fat:4 g, Carbs:6 g, Protein:21 g, Sugars:1 g, Sodium:163.8 mg

Salmon and Cauliflower Mix

Prep time: 10 mins | Servings: 4

Ingredients:
- 4 boneless salmon fillets
- 2 tbsps. Coconut aminos
- Black pepper
- 1 sliced big red onion
- ¼ c. coconut sugar
- 1 head separated cauliflower florets
- 2 tbsps. Olive oil

Directions:
1. In a smaller bowl, mix sugar with coconut aminos and whisk.
2. Heat up a pan with half the oil over medium-high heat, add cauliflower and onion, stir and cook for 10 minutes.
3. Put the salmon inside baking dish, drizzle the remainder inside oil, add coconut aminos, toss somewhat, season with black pepper, introduce within the oven and bake at 400 °F for 10 minutes.
4. Divide the salmon along using the cauliflower mix between plates and serve.
5. Enjoy!

Nutritional Information:
Calories: 220, Fat:3 g, Carbs:12 g, Protein:9 g, Sugars:14.9 g, Sodium:757.5 mg

Creamy Salmon and Asparagus Mix

Prep time: 10 mins | Servings: 6

Ingredients:
- 1 lb. trimmed asparagus
- 1 tbsp. fresh lemon juice
- 20 oz. skinless and deboned salmon
- Black pepper
- 1 Oz. Grated mozzarella, grated
- 1 tbsp. grated lemon zest
- 1 c. coconut cream

Directions:
1. Put some water in the pot, put in a very pinch of salt, bring to your boil over medium heat, add asparagus, cook for 1 minute, transfer for a bowl filled up with ice water, drain and hang up in the bowl.
2. Heat inside pot with the water again over medium heat, add salmon, cook for 5 minutes and in addition drain.
3. In a bowl, mix lemon peel with cream and lemon juice and whisk
4. 4.Heat up a pan over medium-high heat, asparagus, cream and pepper, cook for 1 more minute, divide between plates, add salmon and serve with grated parmesan.
5. Enjoy!

Nutritional Information:
Calories: 354, Fat:2 g, Carbs:2 g, Protein:4 g, Sugars:1.1 g, Sodium:204.5 mg

Salmon in Dill Sauce

Prep time: 10 mins | Servings: 6

Ingredients:
- 6 salmon fillets
- 1 c. low-fat, low-sodium chicken broth
- 1 tsp. cayenne pepper
- 2 tbsps. Fresh lemon juice
- 2 c. water
- ¼ c. chopped fresh dill

Directions:
1. In a slow cooker, mix together water, broth, lemon juice, lemon juice and dill.
2. Arrange salmon fillets on top, skin side down.
3. Sprinkle with cayenne pepper.
4. Set the slow cooker on low.
5. Cover and cook for about 1-2 hours.

Nutritional Information:
Calories: 360, Fat:8 g, Carbs:44 g, Protein:28 g, Sugars:0.5 g, Sodium:8 mg

Easy Salmon and Brussels Sprouts

Prep time: 10 mins | Servings: 6

Ingredients:
- 6 deboned medium salmon fillets
- 1 tsp. onion powder
- 1 ¼ lbs. halved Brussels sprouts
- 3 tbsps. Extra virgin extra virgin olive oil
- 2 tbsps. Brown sugar
- 1 tsp. garlic powder
- 1 tsp. smoked paprika

Directions:
1. In a bowl, mix sugar with onion powder, garlic powder, smoked paprika as well as a number of tablespoon olive oil and whisk well.
2. Spread Brussels sprouts about the lined baking sheet, drizzle the rest in the essential extra virgin olive oil, toss to coat, introduce in the oven at 450 °F and bake for 5 minutes.
3. Add salmon fillets brush with sugar mix you've prepared, introduce inside the oven and bake for 15 minutes more.
4. Divide everything between plates and serve.
5. Enjoy!

Nutritional Information:
Calories: 212, Fat:5 g, Carbs:12 g, Protein:8 g, Sugars:3.7 g, Sodium:299.1 mg

Shrimp Lo Mein

Prep time: 10 mins | Servings: 6

Ingredients:
- 1 tbsp. cornstarch
- 1 lb. medium-size frozen raw shrimp
- 1 c. frozen shelled edamame
- 3 tbsps. Light teriyaki sauce
- 16 Oz. Drained and rinsed tofu spaghetti noodles
- 18 oz. frozen Szechuan vegetable blend with sesame sauce

Directions:
1. Microwave noodles for 1 minute; set aside. Place shrimp in a small bowl and toss with 2 tablespoons teriyaki sauce; set aside.
2. Place mixed vegetables and edamame in a large nonstick skillet with 1/4 cup water. Cover and cook, stirring occasionally, over medium-high heat for 7 minutes or until cooked through.
3. Stir shrimp into vegetable mixture; cover and cook 4 to 5 minutes or until shrimp is pink and cooked through.
4. Stir together remaining 1 tablespoon teriyaki sauce and the cornstarch, then stir into the mixture in the skillet until thickened. Gently stir noodles into skillet and cook until warmed through.

Nutritional Information:
Calories: 252, Fat:7.1 g, Carbs:35.2 g, Protein:12.1 g, Sugars:2.2 g, Sodium:180 mg

Salmon and Potatoes Mix

Prep time: 10 mins | Servings: 4

Ingredients:
- 4 oz. chopped smoked salmon
- 1 tbsp. essential olive oil
- Black pepper
- 1 tbsp. chopped chives
- ¼ c. coconut cream
- 1 ½ lbs. chopped potatoes
- 2 tsps. Prepared horseradish

Directions:
1. Heat up a pan using the oil over medium heat, add potatoes and cook for 10 minutes.
2. Add salmon, chives, horseradish, cream and black pepper, toss, cook for 1 minute more, divide between plates and serve.
3. Enjoy!

Nutritional Information:
Calories: 233, Fat:6 g, Carbs:9 g, Protein:11 g, Sugars:3.3 g, Sodium:97 mg

Smoked Salmon and Radishes

Prep time: 10 mins | Servings: 8

Ingredients:
- ½ c. drained and chopped capers
- 1 lb. skinless, de-boned and flaked smoked salmon
- 4 chopped radishes
- 3 tbsps. Chopped chives
- 3 tbsps. Prepared beet horseradish
- 2 tsps. Grated lemon zest
- 1/3 c. roughly chopped red onion

Directions:
1. In a bowl, combine the salmon while using the beet horseradish, lemon zest, radish, capers, onions and chives, toss and serve cold.
2. Enjoy!

Nutritional Information:
Calories: 254, Fat:2 g, Carbs:7 g, Protein:7 g, Sugars:1.4 g, Sodium:660 mg

Parmesan Baked Fish

Prep time: 10 mins | Servings: 4

Ingredients:
- ½ tsp. Worcestershire sauce
- 1/3 c. mayonnaise
- 3 tbsps. Freshly grated parmesan cheese
- 4 oz. cod fish fillets
- 1 tbsp. snipped fresh chives

Directions:
1. Preheat oven to 450°C.
2. Rinse fish and pat dry with paper towels; spray an 8x8x2" baking dish with non-stick pan spray, set aside.
3. In small bowl stir mayo, grated cheese, chives, and Worcestershire sauce; spread mixture over fish fillets.
4. Bake, uncovered, 12-15 minutes or until fish flakes easily with a fork

Nutritional Information:
Calories:850.5 , Fat: 24.8g, Carbs:44.5 g, Protein:104.6 g, Sugars:0.6 g, Sodium:307.7 mg

Shrimp and Mango Mix

Prep time: 10 mins | Servings: 4

Ingredients:
- 3 tbsps. Finely chopped parsley
- 3 tbsps. Coconut sugar
- 1 lb. peeled, deveined and cooked shrimp
- 6 tbsps. Avocado mayonnaise
- 3 tbsps. Balsamic vinegar
- 3 peeled and cubed mangos

Directions:
1. In a bowl, mix vinegar with sugar and mayo and whisk.
2. In another bowl, combine the mango with the parsley and shrimp, add the mayo mix, toss and serve.
3. Enjoy!

Nutritional Information:
Calories: 204 , Fat: 3 g, Carbs: 8 g, Protein: 8 g, Sugars: 12.6 g, Sodium: 273.4 mg

Roasted Hake

Prep time: 20 mins | Servings: 4

Ingredients:
- ½ c. tomato sauce
- 2 sliced tomatoes
- Fresh parsley
- ½ c. grated cheese
- 4 lbs. deboned hake fish
- 1 tbsp. olive oil
- Salt.

Directions:

1. Season the fish with salt. Pan-fry the fish until half-done.
2. Shape foil into containers according to the number of fish pieces.
3. Pour tomato sauce into each foil dish; arrange the fish, then the tomato slices, again add tomato sauce and sprinkle with grated cheese.
4. Bake in the oven at 400 F until there is a golden crust.
5. Serve with fresh parsley.

Nutritional Information:
Calories: 421, Fat:48.7 g, Carbs:2.4 g, Protein:17.4 g, Sugars:0.5 g, Sodium:94.6 mg

Coconut Cream Shrimp

Prep time: 10 mins | Servings: 2

Ingredients:
- 1 tbsp. coconut cream
- ½ tsp. lime juice
- ¼ tsp. black pepper
- 1 tbsp. parsley
- 1 lb. cooked, peeled and deveined shrimp
- ¼ tsp. chopped jalapeno

Directions:
1. In a bowl, mix the shrimp while using cream, jalapeno, lime juice, parsley and black pepper, toss, divide into small bowls and serve.
2. Enjoy!

Nutritional Information:
Calories: 183, Fat:5 g, Carbs:12 g, Protein:8 g, Sugars:0.9 g, Sodium:474.9 mg

Simple Cinnamon Salmon

Prep time: 10 mins | Servings: 2

Ingredients:
- 1 tbsp. organic essential olive oil
- Black pepper
- 1 tbsp. cinnamon powder
- 2 de-boned salmon fillets

Directions:
1. Heat up a pan with the oil over medium heat, add pepper and cinnamon and stir well.
2. Add salmon, skin side up, cook for 5 minutes on both sides, divide between plates and serve by using a side salad.
3. Enjoy!

Nutritional Information:
Calories: 220, Fat:8 g, Carbs:11 g, Protein:8 g, Sugars:9.3 g, Sodium:250.5 mg

Lemon-Herb Grilled Fish

Prep time: 5 mins | Servings: 4

Ingredients:
- 4 peeled garlic cloves
- ¼ tsp. salt
- 8 lemon slices
- ¼ tsp. ground black pepper
- Remoulade
- 2 small blue-fish
- 2 sprigs fresh thyme

Directions:
1. Prepare outdoor grill with medium-low to medium coals, or heat gas grill to medium-low to medium (to broil, see Note below).
2. Rinse fish; pat dry. Cut 3 slashes on each side. Season with salt, pepper.
3. Stuff 3 lemon slices in cavity of each fish. Add thyme and 2 cloves garlic to each cavity.
4. Grill fish 6 inches from heat, covered, 10 to 12 minutes, until just beginning to char. Flip over carefully. Cover each eye with one of remaining lemon slices. Grill 12 to 15 minutes more, until flesh is white throughout.
5. Transfer fish to platter. For each, pry up top fillet in one piece, flipping over, and skin side down.

6. Beginning at tail, carefully pull up end of spine of fish, and lift up, removing whole backbone. Remove any small bones from fish.
7. Serve with Remoulade.

Nutritional Information:
Calories: 118.1, Fat:6.8 g, Carbs:1 g, Protein:12.9 g, Sugars:12.9 g, Sodium:91.2 mg

Scallops and Strawberry Mix

Prep time: 20 mins | Servings: 2

Ingredients:
- 1 tbsp. lime juice
- ½ c. Pico de gallo
- Black pepper
- 4 oz. scallops
- ½ c. chopped strawberries

Directions:
1. Heat up a pan over medium heat, add scallops, cook for 3 minutes on both sides and take away heat,
2. In a bowl, mix strawberries with lime juice, Pico de gallo, scallops and pepper, toss and serve cold.
3. Enjoy!

Nutritional Information:
Calories: 169, Fat:2 g, Carbs:8 g, Protein:13 g, Sugars:0 g, Sodium:235.7 mg

Cod Peas Relish

Prep time: 18-20 mins | Servings: 4-5

Ingredients:
- 1 c. peas
- 2 tbsps. Capers
- 4 de-boned medium cod fillets
- 3 tbsps. Olive oil
- ¼ tsp. black pepper
- 2 tbsps. Lime juice
- 2 tbsps. Chopped shallots
- 1 ½ tbsps. Chopped oregano

Directions:
1. Heat up 1 tbsp. olive oil in a saucepan over medium flame
2. Add the fillets, cook for 5 minutes on each side; set aside.
3. In a bowl of large size, thoroughly mix the oregano, shallots, lime juice, peas, capers, black pepper, and 2 tbsp. olive oil.
4. Toss and serve with the cooked fish.

Nutritional Information:
Calories: 224, Fat:11 g, Carbs:7 g, Protein:24 g, Sugars:2 g, Sodium:485 mg

Chipotle Spiced Shrimp

Prep time: 10 mins | Servings: 4

Ingredients:
- ½ tsp. minced garlic
- 2 tbsps. Tomato paste
- ½ tsp. chopped fresh oregano
- 1 ½ tsps. Water
- ¾ lb. peeled, deveined and uncooked shrimp
- ½ tsp. chipotle chili powder
- ½ tsp. extra-virgin olive oil

Directions:
1. In cold water, rinse shrimp.
2. Pat dry with a paper towel. Set aside on a plate.
3. Whisk together the tomato paste, water and oil in a small bowl to make the marinade. Add garlic, chili powder and oregano and mix well.
4. Spread the marinade (it will be thick) on both sides of the shrimp using a brush and place in the refrigerator.

5. Heat a gas grill or broiler, or prepare a hot fire in a charcoal grill.
6. Coat the grill rack or broiler pan with cooking spray lightly.
7. Put the cooking rack 4 to 6 inches from the heat source.
8. Thread the shrimp onto skewers or lay them in a grill basket, to place on the grill.
9. After 3 to 4 minutes turn the shrimp.
10. When the shrimp is fully cooked, take it off the heat and serve immediately.

Nutritional Information:
Calories: 151.9, Fat:2.8 g, Carbs:5.1 g, Protein:24.2 g, Sugars:2.3 g, Sodium:283.1 mg

Baked Haddock

Prep time: 10 mins | Servings: 4

Ingredients:
- 1 tsp. chopped dill
- 3 tsps. Water
- ¼ tsp. black pepper and salt
- Cooking spray
- 1 lb. chopped haddock
- 2 tbsps. Fresh lemon juice
- 2 tbsps. Avocado mayonnaise

Directions:
1. Spray a baking dish with a few oil, add fish, water, freshly squeezed lemon juice, salt, black pepper, mayo and dill, toss, introduce inside the oven and bake at 350 °F for the half-hour.
2. Divide between plates and serve.
3. Enjoy!

Nutritional Information:
Calories: 264, Fat:4 g, Carbs:7 g, Protein:12 g, Sugars:0 g, Sodium:71.4 mg

Basil Tilapia

Prep time: 10 mins | Servings: 4

Ingredients:
- ½ c. grated low-fat parmesan
- Black pepper
- ¼ c. essential organic olive oil
- 2 tsps. Dried basil, dried
- 4 de-boned tilapia fillets
- 4 tbsps. Avocado mayonnaise
- 2 tbsps. Lemon juice

Directions:
1. Grease a baking dish with all the current oil, add tilapia fillets, black pepper, spread mayo, basil, drizzle fresh freshly squeezed lemon juice and top while using the parmesan, introduce in preheated broiler and cook over medium-high heat for 5 minutes on both sides.
2. Divide between plates and serve developing a side salad.
3. Enjoy!

Nutritional Information:
Calories: 215, Fat:10 g, Carbs:7 g, Protein:11 g, Sugars:0.1 g, Sodium:15.4 mg

Lemony Mussels

Prep time: 5 mins | Servings: 4

Ingredients:
- 1 tbsp. extra virgin extra virgin olive oil
- 2 minced garlic cloves
- 2 lbs. scrubbed mussels
- Juice of one lemon

Directions:
1. Put some water in a pot, add mussels, bring with a boil over medium heat, cook for 5 minutes, discard unopened mussels and transfer them with a bowl.

2. In another bowl, mix the oil with garlic and freshly squeezed lemon juice, whisk well, and add over the mussels, toss and serve.
3. Enjoy!

Nutritional Information:
Calories: 140, Fat:4 g, Carbs:8 g, Protein:8 g, Sugars: 4g, Sodium:600 mg,

Hot Tuna Steak

Prep time: 10 mins | Servings: 6

Ingredients:
- 2 tbsps. Fresh lemon juice
- Pepper.
- Roasted orange garlic mayonnaise
- ¼ c. whole black peppercorns
- 6 sliced tuna steaks
- 2 tbsps. Extra-virgin olive oil
- Salt

Directions:
1. Place the tuna in a bowl to fit. Add the oil, lemon juice, salt and pepper. Turn the tuna to coat well in the marinade. Let rest 15 to 20 minutes, turning once.
2. Place the peppercorns in a double thickness of plastic bags. Tap the peppercorns with a heavy saucepan or small mallet to crush them coarsely. Place on a large plate.
3. When ready to cook the tuna, dip the edges into the crushed peppercorns. Heat a nonstick skillet over medium heat. Sear the tuna steaks, in batches if necessary, for 4 minutes per side for medium-rare fish, adding 2 to 3 tablespoons of the marinade to the skillet if necessary to prevent sticking.
4. Serve dolloped with roasted orange garlic mayonnaise

Nutritional Information:
Calories: 124, Fat:0.4 g, Carbs:0.6 g, Protein:28 g, Sugars:0 g, Sodium:77 mg

Spicy Baked Fish

Prep time: 5 mins | Servings: 5

Ingredients:
- 1 tbsp. olive oil
- 1 tsp. spice salt free seasoning
- 1 lb. salmon fillet

Directions:
1. Preheat the oven to 350F.
2. Sprinkle the fish with olive oil and the seasoning.
3. Bake for 15 min uncovered.
4. Slice and serve.

Nutritional Information:
Calories: 192, Fat:11 g, Carbs:14.9 g, Protein:33.1 g, Sugars:0.3 g, Sodium:505.6 mg

Marinated Fish Steaks

Prep time: 10 mins | Servings: 4

Ingredients:
- 4 lime wedges
- 2 tbsps. Lime juice
- 2 minced garlic cloves
- 2 tsps. Olive oil
- 1 tbsp. snipped fresh oregano
- 1 lb. fresh swordfish
- 1 tsp. lemon-pepper seasoning

Directions:
1. Rinse fish steaks; pat dry with paper towels. Cut into four serving size pieces, if necessary.
2. In a shallow dish combine lime juice, oregano, oil, lemon-pepper seasoning, and garlic. Add fish; turn to coat with marinade.
3. Cover and marinate in refrigerator for 30 minutes to 1-1/2 hours, turning steaks occasionally. Drain fish, reserving marinade.

4. Place fish on the greased unheated rack of a broiler pan.
5. Broil 4 inches from the heat for 8 to 12 minutes or until fish begins to flake when tested with a fork, turning once and brushing with reserved marinade halfway through cooking. Discard any remaining marinade.
6. Before serving, squeeze the juice from one lime wedge over each steak.

Nutritional Information:
Calories: 240, Fat:6 g, Carbs:19 g, Protein:12 g, Sugars:3.27 g, Sodium:325 mg

Baked Tomato Hake

Prep time: 35-40 mins | Servings: 4-5

Ingredients:
- ½ c. tomato sauce
- 1 tbsp. olive oil
- Parsley
- 2 sliced tomatoes
- ½ c. grated cheese
- 4 lbs. de-boned and sliced hake fish
- Salt.

Directions:
1. Preheat the oven to 400 °F.
2. Season the fish with salt.
3. In a skillet or saucepan; stir-fry the fish in the olive oil until half-done.
4. Take four foil papers to cover the fish.
5. Shape the foil to resemble containers; add the tomato sauce into each foil container.
6. Add the fish, tomato slices, and top with grated cheese.
7. Bake until you get a golden crust, for approximately 20-25 minutes.
8. Open the packs and top with parsley.

Nutritional Information:
Calories: 265, Fat:15 g, Carbs:18 g, Protein:22 g, Sugars:0.5 g, Sodium:94.6 mg

Cheesy Tuna Pasta

Prep time: 5-8 min | Servings: 3-4

Ingredients:
- 2 c. arugula
- ¼ c. chopped green onions
- 1 tbs. red vinegar
- 5 oz. drained canned tuna
- ¼ tsp. black pepper
- 2 oz. cooked whole-wheat pasta
- 1 tbsp. olive oil
- 1 tbsp. grated low-fat parmesan

Directions:
1. Cook the pasta in unsalted water until ready. Drain and set aside.
2. In a bowl of large size, thoroughly mix the tuna, green onions, vinegar, oil, arugula, pasta, and black pepper.
3. Toss well and top with the cheese.
4. Serve and enjoy.

Nutritional Information:
Calories: 566.3, Fat:42.4 g, Carbs:18.6 g, Protein:29.8 g, Sugars:0.4 g, Sodium:688.6 mg

Herb-Coated Baked Cod with Honey

Prep time: 5 mins | Servings: 2

Ingredients:
- 6 tbsps. Herb-flavored stuffing
- 8 oz. cod fillets
- 2 tbsps. Honey

Directions:
1. Preheat your oven to 375 °F.
2. Spray a baking pan lightly with cooking spray.
3. Put the herb-flavored stuffing in a bag and close. Squash the stuffing until it gets crumbly.

4. Coat the fishes with honey and get rid of the remaining honey. Add one fillet to the bag of stuffing and shake gently to coat the fish completely.
5. Transfer the cod to the baking pan and repeat the process for the second fish.
6. Wrap the fillets with foil and bake until firm and opaque all through when you test with the tip of a knife blade, about ten minutes.
7. Serve hot.

Nutritional Information:
Calories: 185, Fat:1 g, Carbs:23 g, Protein:21 g, Sugars:2 g, Sodium:144.3 mg

Tender Salmon in Mustard Sauce

Prep time: 10 mins | Servings: 2

Ingredients:
- 5 tbsps. Minced dill
- 2/3 c. sour cream
- Pepper.
- 2 tbsps. Dijon mustard
- 1 tsp. garlic powder
- 5 oz. salmon fillets
- 2-3 tbsps. Lemon juice

Directions:
1. Mix sour cream, mustard, lemon juice and dill.
2. Season the fillets with pepper and garlic powder.
3. Arrange the salmon on a baking sheet skin side down and cover with the prepared mustard sauce.
4. Bake for 20 minutes at 390°F.

Nutritional Information:
Calories: 318, Fat:12 g, Carbs:8 g, Protein:40.9 g, Sugars:909.4 g, Sodium:1.4 mg

Broiled White Sea Bass

Prep time: 5 mins | Servings: 2

Ingredients:
- 1 tsp. minced garlic
- Ground black pepper
- 1 tbsp. lemon juice
- 8 oz. white sea bass fillets
- ¼ tsp. salt-free herbed seasoning blend

Directions:
1. Preheat the broiler and position the rack 4 inches from the heat source.
2. Lightly spray a baking pan with cooking spray. Place the fillets in the pan. Sprinkle the lemon juice, garlic, herbed seasoning and pepper over the fillets.
3. Broil until the fish is opaque throughout when tested with a tip of a knife, about 8 to 10 minutes.
4. Serve immediately.

Nutritional Information:
Calories: 114, Fat:2 g, Carbs:2 g, Protein:21 g, Sugars:0.5 g, Sodium:78 mg

Steamed Fish Balls

Prep time: 10 mins | Servings: 2

Ingredients:
- 2 whisked eggs
- 2 tbsps. Rinsed and cooked rice
- Salt.
- 10 oz. minced white fish fillets

Directions:
1. Combine the minced fish with the rice.
2. Add eggs, season with salt and stir well.
3. Form the balls. Arrange in a steamer basket.
4. Place the basket in a pot with 1 inch of water.
5. Steam, covered, for 30 minutes or until soft.

Nutritional Information:
Calories: 169, Fat:4.3 g, Carbs:1.1 g, Protein:5.3 g, Sugars:0 g, Sodium:173.1 mg

Lemony & Creamy Tilapia

Prep time: 15 mins | Servings: 4

Ingredients:
- 2 tbsps. Chopped fresh cilantro
- ¼ c. low-fat mayonnaise
- Freshly ground black pepper
- ¼ c. fresh lemon juice
- 4 tilapia fillets
- ½ c. grated low-fat parmesan cheese
- ½ tsp. garlic powder

Directions:
1. In a bowl, mix together all ingredients except tilapia fillets and cilantro.
2. Coat the fillets with mayonnaise mixture evenly.
3. Place the filets onto a large foil paper. Wrap the foil paper around fillets to seal them.
4. Arrange the foil packet in the bottom of a large slow cooker.
5. Set the slow cooker on low.
6. Cover and cook for 3-4 hours.
7. Serve with the garnishing of cilantro.

Nutritional Information:
Calories: 133.6, Fat:2.4 g, Carbs:4.6 g, Protein:22 g, Sugars:0.9 g, Sodium:510.4 mg

Smoked Trout Spread

Prep time: 5 mins | Servings: 2

Ingredients:
- 2 tsps. Fresh lemon juice
- ½ c. low-fat cottage cheese
- 1 diced celery stalk
- ¼ lb. skinned smoked trout fillet,
- ½ tsp. Worcestershire sauce
- 1 tsp. hot pepper sauce
- ¼ c. coarsely chopped red onion

Directions:
1. Combine the trout, cottage cheese, red onion, lemon juice, hot pepper sauce and Worcestershire sauce in a blender or food processor.
2. Process until smooth, stopping to scrape down the sides of the bowl as needed.
3. Fold in the diced celery.
4. Keep in an air-tight container in the refrigerator.

Nutritional Information:
Calories: 57, Fat:4 g, Carbs:1 g, Protein:4 g, Sugars:0 g, Sodium:660 mg

Broiled Sea Bass

Prep time: 10 mins | Servings: 2

Ingredients:
- 2 minced garlic cloves
- Pepper.
- 1 tbsp. lemon juice
- 2 white sea bass fillets
- ¼ tsp. herb seasoning blend

Directions:
1. Spray a broiler pan with some olive oil and place the fillets on it.
2. Sprinkle the lemon juice, garlic and the spices over the fillets.
3. Broil for about 10 min or until the fish is golden.
4. Serve over a bed of sautéed spinach if desired.

Nutritional Information:
Calories: 169, Fat:9.3 g, Carbs:0.34 g, Protein:15.3 g, Sugars:0.2 g, Sodium:323 mg

Spicy Cod

Prep time: 29 mins | Servings: 4

Ingredients:
- 2 tbsps. Fresh chopped parsley
- 2 lbs. cod fillets
- 2 c. low sodium salsa
- 1 tbsp. flavorless oil

Directions:
1. Preheat the oven to 350°F.

2. In a large, deep baking dish drizzle the oil along the bottom. Place the cod fillets in the dish. Pour the salsa over the fish. Cover with foil for 20 minutes. Remove the foil last 10 minutes of cooking.
3. Bake in the oven for 20 – 30 minutes, until the fish is flaky.
4. Serve with white or brown rice. Garnish with parsley.

Nutritional Information:
Calories: 110, Fat:11 g, Carbs:83 g, Protein:16.5 g, Sugars:0 g, Sodium:122 mg

Lemon Salmon with Kaffir Lime

Prep time: 40 mins | Servings: 8

Ingredients:
- 1 quartered and bruised lemon grass stalk
- 2 kaffir torn lime leaves
- 1 thinly sliced lemon
- 1 ½ c. fresh coriander leaves
- 1 whole side salmon fillet

Directions:
1. Pre-heat the oven to 350°F.
2. Cover a baking pan with foil sheets, overlapping the sides
3. Place the Salmon on the foil, top with the lemon, lime leaves, the lemon grass and 1 cup of the coriander leaves. Option: season with salt and pepper.
4. Bring the long side of foil to the center before folding the seal. Roll the ends in order to close up the salmon.
5. Bake for 30 minutes.
6. Transfer the cooked fish to a platter. Top with fresh coriander. Serve with white or brown rice.

Nutritional Information:
Calories: 103, Fat:11.8 g, Carbs:43.5 g, Protein:18 g, Sugars:0.7 g, Sodium:322 mg

Heartfelt Tuna Melt

Prep time: 10 mins | Servings: 4

Ingredients:
- 3 oz. grated reduced-fat cheddar cheese
- 1/3 c. chopped celery
- Black pepper and salt
- ¼ c. chopped onion
- 2 whole-wheat English muffins
- 6 oz. drained white tuna
- ¼ c. low fat Russian

Directions:
1. Preheat broiler. Combine tuna, celery, onion and salad dressing.
2. Season with salt and pepper.
3. Toast English muffin halves.
4. Place split-side-up on baking sheet and top each with 1/4 of tuna mixture.
5. Broil 2-3 minutes or until heated through.
6. Top with cheese and return to broiler until cheese is melted, about 1 minute longer.

Nutritional Information:
Calories: 320, Fat:16.7 g, Carbs:17.1 g, Protein:25.7 g, Sugars:5.85 g, Sodium:832 mg

Crab Salad

Prep time: 10 mins | Servings: 4

Ingredients:
- 2 c. crab meat
- 1 c. halved cherry tomatoes
- 1 tbsp. olive oil
- Black pepper
- 1 chopped shallot
- 1/3 c. chopped cilantro
- 1 tbsp. lemon juice

Directions:
1. In a bowl, combine the crab with the tomatoes and the other ingredients, toss and serve.

Nutritional Information:
Calories: 54, Fat:3.9 g, Carbs:2.6 g, Protein:2.3 g, Sugars:2.3 g, Sodium:462.5 mg

Minty Cod Mix

Prep time: 10 mins | Servings: 4

Ingredients:
- 4 boneless cod fillets
- ½ c. low-sodium chicken stock
- 2 tbsps. olive oil
- ¼ tsp. black pepper
- 1 tbsp. chopped mint
- 1 tsps. grated lemon zest
- ¼ c. chopped shallot
- 1 tbsp. lemon juice

Directions:
1. Heat up a pan with the oil over medium heat, add the shallots, stir and sauté for 5 minutes.
2. Add the cod, the lemon juice and the other ingredients, bring to a simmer and cook over medium heat for 12 minutes.
3. Divide everything between plates and serve.

Nutritional Information:
Calories: 160, Fat:8.1 g, Carbs:2 g, Protein:20.5 g, Sugars:8 g, Sodium:45 mg

Salmon and Dill Capers

Prep time: 10 mins | Servings: 4

Ingredients:
- 1 tbsp. drained capers
- 2 tbsps. olive oil
- 1 tbsp. chopped dill
- ½ c. coconut cream
- ¼ tsp. black pepper
- 4 boneless salmon fillets
- 1 chopped shallot

Directions:
1. Heat up a pan with the oil over medium-high heat, add the shallot and the capers, toss and sauté for 4 minutes.
2. Add the salmon and cook it for 3 minutes on each side.
3. Add the rest of the ingredients, cook everything for 5 minutes more, divide between plates and serve.

Nutritional Information:
Calories: 369, Fat:25.2 g, Carbs:2.7 g, Protein:35.5g, Sugars:0.1 g, Sodium:311.2 mg

Creamy Sea Bass Mix

Prep time: 10 mins | Servings: 4

Ingredients:
- 1 tbsp. chopped parsley
- 2 tbsps. avocado oil
- 1 c. coconut cream
- 1 tbsp. lime juice
- 1 chopped yellow onion
- ¼ tsp. black pepper
- 4 boneless sea bass fillets

Directions:
1. Heat up a pan with the oil over medium heat, add the onion, toss and sauté for 2 minutes.
2. Add the fish and cook it for 4 minutes on each side.
3. Add the rest of the ingredients, cook everything for 4 minutes more, divide between plates and serve.

Nutritional Information:
Calories: 283, Fat:12.3 g, Carbs:12.5 g, Protein:8 g, Sugars:6 g, Sodium:508.8 mg

Tuna and Shallots

Prep time: 10 mins | Servings: 4

Ingredients:
- ½ c. low-sodium chicken stock
- 1 tbsp. olive oil
- 4 boneless and skinless tuna fillets
- 2 chopped shallots
- 1 tsp. sweet paprika
- 2 tbsps. lime juice

- ¼ tsp. black pepper

Directions:
1. Heat up a pan with the oil over medium-high heat, add shallots and sauté for 3 minutes.
2. Add the fish and cook it for 4 minutes on each side.
3. Add the rest of the ingredients, cook everything for 3 minutes more, divide between plates and serve.

Nutritional Information:
Calories: 4040, Fat:34.6 g, Carbs:3 g, Protein:21.4 g, Sugars:0.5 g, Sodium:1000 mg

Paprika Tuna

Prep time: 4 mins | Servings: 4

Ingredients:
- ½ tsp. chili powder
- 2 tsps. sweet paprika
- ¼ tsp. black pepper
- 2 tbsps. olive oil
- 4 boneless tuna steaks

Directions:
1. Heat up a pan with the oil over medium-high heat, add the tuna steaks, season with paprika, black pepper and chili powder, cook for 5 minutes on each side, divide between plates and serve with a side salad.

Nutritional Information:
Calories: 455, Fat:20.6 g, Carbs:0.8 g, Protein:63.8 g, Sugars:7.4 g, Sodium: 411 mg

Ginger Sea Bass Mix

Prep time: 10 mins | Servings: 4

Ingredients:
- 4 boneless sea bass fillets
- 2 tbsps. olive oil
- 1 tsp. grated ginger
- 1 tbsp. chopped cilantro
- Black pepper
- 1 tbsp. balsamic vinegar

Directions:
1. Heat up a pan with the oil over medium heat, add the fish and cook for 5 minutes on each side.
2. Add the rest of the ingredients, cook everything for 5 minutes more, divide everything between plates and serve.

Nutritional Information:
Calories: 267, Fat:11.2 g, Carbs:1.5 g, Protein:23 g, Sugars:0.78 g, Sodium:321.2 mg

Parmesan Cod Mix

Prep time: 10 mins | Servings: 4

Ingredients:
- 1 tbsp. lemon juice
- ½ c. chopped green onion
- 4 boneless cod fillets
- 3 minced garlic cloves
- 1 tbsp. olive oil
- ½ c. shredded low-fat parmesan cheese

Directions:
1. Heat up a pan with the oil over medium heat, add the garlic and the green onions, toss and sauté for 5 minutes.
2. Add the fish and cook it for 4 minutes on each side.
3. Add the lemon juice, sprinkle the parmesan on top, cook everything for 2 minutes more, divide between plates and serve.

Nutritional Information:
Calories: 275, Fat:22.1 g, Carbs:18.2 g, Protein:12 g, Sugars:0.34 g, Sodium:285.4 mg

Chapter 6 Beef, Pork and Lamb

Authentic Pepper Steak

Prep time: 5 mins | Servings: 4

Ingredients:
- 1 tbsp. sesame oil
- 80 oz. sliced mushroom
- 1 c. water
- 1 sliced red pepper piece
- 1 pack onion soup mix
- 1 lb. de-boned beef eye of round steak
- 1 tbsp. minced garlic

Directions:
1. Add the listed ingredients to your Instant Pot
2. Lock up the lid and cook on HIGH pressure for 20 minutes
3. Release the pressure naturally over 10 minutes
4. Serve the pepper steak and enjoy!

Nutritional Information:
Calories: 222, Fat:15 g, Carbs:5 g, Protein:36 g, Sugars:1.56 g, Sodium:556 mg

Lamb Chops with Rosemary

Prep time: 5 mins | Servings: 4

Ingredients:
- 1 lb. lamb chops
- ½ tsp. freshly ground black pepper
- 1 tbsp. olive oil
- 5 garlic cloves
- 1 tbsp. chopped fresh rosemary

Directions:
1. Adjust oven rack to the top third of the oven. Preheat broiler. Line a baking sheet with foil.
2. Place the garlic, rosemary, pepper, and olive oil into a small bowl and stir well to combine.
3. Place the lamb chops on a baking sheet and brush half of the garlic-rosemary mixture equally between the chops, coating well. Place the sheet beneath broiler and broil 4–5 minutes.
4. Remove from oven and carefully flip over the chops. Divide the remaining garlic-rosemary mixture evenly between the chops and spread to coat. Return pan to oven and broil for another 3 minutes.
5. Remove from oven and serve immediately.

Nutritional Information:
Calories: 185, Fat:9 g, Carbs:1 g, Protein:23 g, Sugars:0 g, Sodium:72.8 mg

Cane Wrapped Around In Prosciutto

Prep time: 3 mins | Servings: 4

Ingredients:
- 80 oz. sliced prosciutto
- 1 lb. thick asparagus

Directions:
1. The first step here is to prepare your instant pot by pouring in about 2 cups of water
2. Take the asparagus and wrap them up in prosciutto spears.
3. Once all of the asparagus are wrapped, gently place the processed asparaguses in the cooking basket inside your pot in layers.
4. Turn up the heat to a high temperature and when there is a pressure build up, take down the heat and let it cook for about 2-3 minutes at the high pressure.
5. Once the timer runs out, gently open the cover of the pressure cooker
6. Take out the steamer basket from the pot instantly and toss the asparaguses on a plate to serve
7. Eat warm or let them come down to room temperature

Nutritional Information:
Calories: 212, Fat:14 g, Carbs:11 g, Protein:12 g, Sugars:367.6 g, Sodium:0 mg

Beef Veggie Pot Meal

Prep time: 45-50 mins | Servings: 2-3

Ingredients:
- 1 tsp. butter
- ¼ shredded cabbage head
- 2 peeled and sliced carrots
- 1 tbsp. flour
- 4 tbsps. sour cream
- 1 chopped onion
- 10 oz. sliced and boiled beef tenderloin

Directions:
1. In a saucepan; add the butter, cabbage, carrots, and onions.
2. Cook on medium-high heat until the veggies get softened.
3. Add the beef meat and stir the mix.
4. In a mixing bowl, beat the cream with flour until smooth.
5. Add the sauce over the beef.
6. Cover and cook for 40 minutes.
7. Serve warm.

Nutritional Information:
Calories: 245.5, Fat:10.2 g, Carbs:18.4 g, Protein:19.0 g, Sugars:5.5 g, Sodium:188.2 mg

Braised Beef Shanks

Prep time: 10 mins | Servings: 2

Ingredients:
- Freshly ground black pepper
- 5 minced garlic cloves
- 1½ lbs. lean beef shanks
- 2 sprigs fresh rosemary
- 1 c. low-fat, low-sodium beef broth
- 1 tbsp. fresh lime juice

Directions:
1. In a slow cooker, add all ingredients and mix.
2. Set the slow cooker on low.
3. Cover and cook for 4-6 hours.

Nutritional Information:
Calories: 50, Fat:1 g, Carbs:0.8 g, Protein:8 g, Sugars:0 g, Sodium:108 mg

Beef Heart

Prep time: 40 mins | Servings: 4

Ingredients:
- 1 chopped large onion
- 1 c. water
- 2 peeled and chopped tomatoes
- 1 boiled beef heart
- 2 tbsps. tomato paste

Directions:
1. Boil the beef heart until half-done.
2. Sauté the onions with tomatoes until soft.
3. Cut the beef heart into cubes and add to tomato and onion mixture. Add water and tomato paste. Stew on low heat for 30 minutes.

Nutritional Information:
Calories: 138, Fat:3 g, Carbs:0.1 g, Protein:24.2 g, Sugars:0 g, Sodium:50.2 mg

Beef with Mushrooms

Prep time: 15 mins | Servings: 8

Ingredients:
- 2 c. salt-free tomato paste
- 2 c. sliced fresh mushrooms
- 2 c. low-fat, low-sodium beef broth
- 2 lbs. cubed lean beef stew meat
- 1 c. chopped fresh parsley leaves
- Freshly ground black pepper
- 4 minced garlic cloves

Directions:

1. In a slow cooker add all ingredients except lemon juice and, stir to combine.
2. Set the slow cooker on low.
3. Cover and cook for about 8 hours.
4. Serve hot with the drizzling of lemon juice

Nutritional Information:
Calories: 260, Fat:12 g, Carbs:18 g, Protein:44 g, Sugars:4 g, Sodium:480 mg

Lemony Braised Beef Roast

Prep time: 15 mins | Servings: 6

Ingredients:
- 1 tbsp. minced fresh rosemary
- ½ c. low-fat, low-sodium beef broth
- Freshly ground black pepper
- 2 lbs. lean beef pot roast
- 1 sliced onion
- 2 minced garlic cloves
- ¼ c. fresh lemon juice
- 1 tsp. ground cumin

Directions:
1. In a large slow cooker, add all ingredients and mix well.
2. Set the slow cooker on low.
3. Cover and cook for about 6-8 hours.

Nutritional Information:
Calories: 344, Fat:2.8 g, Carbs:18 g, Protein:32 g, Sugars:2.4 g, Sodium:278 mg

Grilled Fennel-Cumin Lamb Chops

Prep time: 10 mins | Servings: 2

Ingredients:
- ¼ tsp. salt
- 1 minced large garlic clove
- 1/8 tsp. cracked black pepper
- ¾ tsp. crushed fennel seeds
- ¼ tsp. ground coriander
- 4-6 sliced lamb rib chops
- ¾ tsp. ground cumin

Directions:
1. Trim fat from chops. Place the chops on a plate.
2. In a small bowl combine the garlic, fennel seeds, cumin, salt, coriander, and black pepper. Sprinkle the mixture evenly over chops; rub in with your fingers. Cover the chops with plastic wrap and marinate in the refrigerator at least 30 minutes or up to 24 hours.
3. Grill chops on the rack of an uncovered grill directly over medium coals until chops are desired doneness.

Nutritional Information:
Calories: 239, Fat:12 g, Carbs:2 g, Protein:29 g, Sugars:0 g, Sodium:409 mg

Jerk Beef and Plantain Kabobs

Prep time: 10 mins | Servings: 4

Ingredients:
- 2 peeled and sliced ripe plantains
- 2 tbsps. Red wine vinegar
- Lime wedges
- 1 tbsp. cooking oil
- 1 sliced medium red onion
- 12 oz. sliced boneless beef sirloin steak
- 1 tbsp. Jamaican jerk seasoning

Directions:
1. Trim fat from meat. Cut into 1-inch pieces. In a small bowl, stir together red wine vinegar, oil, and jerk seasoning. Toss meat cubes with half of the vinegar mixture. On long skewers, alternately thread meat, plantain chunks, and onion wedges, leaving a 1/4-inch space between pieces.

2. Brush plantains and onion wedges with remaining vinegar mixture.
3. Place skewers on the rack of an uncovered grill directly over medium coals. Grill for 12 to 15 minutes or until meat is desired doneness, turning occasionally.
4. Serve with lime wedges.

Nutritional Information:
Calories: 260, Fat:7 g, Carbs:21 g, Protein:26 g, Sugars:2.5 g, Sodium:358 mg

Beef Pot

Prep time: 10 mins | Servings: 2

Ingredients:
- 4 tbsps. Sour cream
- ¼ shredded cabbage head
- 1 tsp. butter
- 2 peeled and sliced carrots
- 1 chopped onion
- 10 oz. boiled and sliced beef tenderloin
- 1 tbsp. flour

Directions:
1. Sauté the cabbage, carrots and onions in butter.
2. Spray a pot with cooking spray.
3. In layers place the sautéed vegetables, then beef, then another layer of vegetables.
4. Beat the sour cream with flour until smooth and pour over the beef.
5. Cover and bake at 400F for 40 minutes.

Nutritional Information:
Calories: 210, Fat:30 g, Carbs:4 g, Protein:14 g, Sugars:1 g, Sodium:600 mg

Beef with Cucumber Raita

Prep time: 10 mins | Servings: 2

Ingredients:
- ½ tsp. lemon-pepper seasoning
- ¼ c. coarsely shredded unpeeled cucumber
- Black pepper and salt
- 1 tbsp. finely chopped red onion
- ¼ tsp. sugar
- 1 lb. sliced de-boned beef sirloin steak
- 8 oz. plain fat-free yogurt
- 1 tbsp. snipped fresh mint

Directions:
1. Preheat broiler.
2. In a small bowl combine yogurt, cucumber, onion, snipped mint, and sugar. Season to taste with salt and pepper; set aside
3. Trim fat from meat. Sprinkle meat with lemon-pepper seasoning.
4. Place meat on the unheated rack of a broiler pan. Broil 3 to 4 inches from heat, turning meat over after half of the broiling time.
5. Allow 15 to 17 minutes for medium-rare (145 degree F) and 20 to 22 minutes for medium (160 degree F).
6. Cut steak across the grain into thin slices.
7. Serve and enjoy.

Nutritional Information:
Calories: 176, Fat:3 g, Carbs:5 g, Protein:28 g, Sugars:8.9 g, Sodium:88.3 mg

Bistro Beef Tenderloin

Prep time: 10 mins | Servings: 12

Ingredients:
- 2 tbsps. Extra-virgin olive oil
- 2 tbsps. Dijon mustard
- 1 tsp. kosher salt
- 2/3 c. chopped mixed fresh herbs
- 3 lbs. trimmed beef tenderloin
- ½ tsp. freshly ground pepper

Directions:
1. Preheat oven to 400 °F.

2. Tie kitchen string around tenderloin in three places so it doesn't flatten while roasting.
3. Rub the tenderloin with oil; pat on salt and pepper. Place in a large roasting pan.
4. Roast until a thermometer inserted into the thickest part of the tenderloin registers 140 °F for medium-rare, about 45 minutes, turning two or three times during roasting to ensure even cooking.
5. Transfer to a cutting board; let rest for 10 minutes. Remove the string.
6. Place herbs on a large plate. Coat the tenderloin evenly with mustard; then roll in the herbs, pressing gently to adhere. Slice and serve.

Nutritional Information:
Calories: 280, Fat:20.6 g, Carbs:0.9 g, Protein:22.2 g, Sugars:0 g, Sodium:160 mg

The Surprising No "Noodle" Lasagna

Prep time: 10 mins | Servings: 8

Ingredients:
- ½ c. parmesan cheese
- 2 minced garlic cloves
- 8 oz. sliced mozzarella
- 1 lb. ground beef
- 25 oz. marinara sauce
- 1 small sized onion
- 1 ½ c. ricotta cheese
- 1 large sized egg

Directions:
1. Set your pot to Sauté mode and add garlic, onion and ground beef
2. Take a small bowl and add ricotta and parmesan with egg and mix
3. Drain the grease and transfer the beef to a 1 and a ½ quart soufflé dish
4. Add marinara sauce to the browned meat and reserve half
5. Top the remaining meat sauce with half of your mozzarella cheese
6. Spread half of the ricotta cheese over the mozzarella layer
7. Top with the remaining meat sauce
8. Add a final layer of mozzarella cheese on top
9. Spread any remaining ricotta cheese mix over the mozzarella
10. Carefully add this mixture to your Soufflé Dish
11. Pour 1 cup of water to your pot
12. Place it over a trivet
13. Lock up the lid and cook on HIGH pressure for 10 minutes
14. Release the pressure naturally over 10 minutes
15. Serve and enjoy!

Nutritional Information:
Calories: 607, Fat:23 g, Carbs:65 g, Protein:33 g, Sugars:0.31 g, Sodium:128 mg

Lamb Chops with Kale

Prep time: 10 mins | Servings: 4

Ingredients:
- 1 tbsp. olive oil
- 1 sliced yellow onion
- 1 c. torn kale
- 2 tbsps. low-sodium tomato paste
- ¼ tsp. black pepper
- ½ c. low-sodium veggie stock
- 1 lb. lamb chops

Directions:
1. Grease a roasting pan with the oil, arrange the lamb chops inside, also add the kale and the other ingredients and toss gently.
2. Bake everything at 390 °F for 35 minutes, divide between plates and serve.

Nutritional Information:
Calories: 275, Fat:11.8 g, Carbs:7.3 g, Protein:33.6 g, Sugars:0.1 g, Sodium:280 mg

Thyme Beef and Potatoes Mix

Prep time: 10 mins | Servings: 4

Ingredients:
- 3 tbsps. olive oil
- ½ lb. ground beef
- 1 c. no-salt-added, and chopped canned tomatoes
- ¼ tsp. black pepper
- 1 ¾ lbs. peeled and roughly cubed red potatoes
- 2 tsps. dried thyme
- 1 chopped yellow onion

Directions:
1. Heat up a pan with the oil over medium-high heat, add the onion and the beef, stir and brown for 5 minutes.
2. Add the potatoes and the rest of the ingredients, toss, bring to a simmer, cook for 20 minutes more, divide into bowls and serve for lunch.

Nutritional Information:
Calories: 216, Fat:14.5 g, Carbs:40.7 g, Protein:22.2 g, Sugars:1 g, Sodium:130 mg

Lamb and Bok Choy Pan

Prep time: 10 mins | Servings: 4

Ingredients:
- 1 chopped carrot
- 1 c. torn bok choy
- 2 tbsps. avocado oil
- 1 chopped yellow onion
- 1 lb. roughly cubed lamb stew meat
- Black pepper
- 1 c. low-sodium chicken stock

Directions:
1. Heat up a pan with the oil over medium-high heat, add the onion and the carrot and sauté for 5 minutes.
2. Add the meat and brown for 5 minutes more.
3. Add the rest of the ingredients, bring to a simmer and cook over medium heat for 20 minutes.
4. Divide everything between plates and serve.

Nutritional Information:
Calories: 360, Fat:14.5 g, Carbs:22.4 g, Protein:16 g, Sugars:2.4 g, Sodium:620 mg

Simple Veal Chops

Prep time: 10 mins | Servings: 4

Ingredients:
- 3 tbsps. essential olive oil
- Zest of 1 grated lemon
- 3 tbsps. whole-wheat flour
- 1 ½ c. whole-wheat breadcrumbs
- Black pepper
- 1 tbsp. milk
- 4 veal rib chops
- 2 eggs

Directions:
1. Put whole-wheat flour within a bowl.
2. In another bowl, mix eggs with milk and whisk
3. In 1 / 3 bowl, mix the breadcrumbs with lemon zest.
4. Season veal chops with black pepper, dredge them in flour, and dip inside egg mix then in breadcrumbs.
5. Heat up a pan because of the oil over medium-high heat, add veal chops, cook for 2 main minutes on both sides and transfer to some baking sheet, introduce them inside oven at 350 ^{0}F, bake for quarter-hour, divide between plates and serve utilizing a side salad.
6. Enjoy!

Nutritional Information:
Calories: 270, Fat:6 g, Carbs:10 g, Protein:16 g, Sugars:0 g, Sodium: 320 mg

Beef & Vegetable Stir-fry

Prep time: 20 mins | Servings: 4

Ingredients:
- 1 lb. thinly sliced skirt steak
- 2 tbsps. sesame seeds
- ¾ c. stir-fry sauce
- 1 thinly sliced red bell pepper
- 2 thinly sliced scallions
- 2 tbsps. canola oil
- ¼ tsp. ground black pepper
- 1 sliced broccoli head
- 1½ c. fluffy brown rice

Directions:
1. Prepare the Stir-Fry Sauce.
2. Heat the canola oil in a large wok or skillet over medium-high heat. Season the steak with the black pepper and cook for 4 minutes, until crispy on the outside and pink on the inside. Remove the steak from the skillet and place the broccoli and peppers in the hot oil. Stir-fry for 4 minutes, stirring or tossing occasionally, until crisp and slightly tender.
3. Place the steak back in the skillet with the vegetables. Pour the stir-fry sauce over the steak and vegetables and let simmer for 3 minutes. Remove from the heat.
4. Serve the stir-fry over rice and top with the scallions and sesame seeds.
5. For leftovers, divide the stir-fry evenly into microwaveable airtight containers and store in the refrigerator for up to 5 days. Reheat in the microwave on high for 2 to 3 minutes, until heated through.

Nutritional Information:
Calories: 408, Fat:18 g, Carbs:36 g, Protein:31 g, Sugars:5.5 g, Sodium:197 mg

Beef and Barley Farmers Soup

Prep time: 10 mins | Servings: 4

Ingredients:
- 1 diced onion
- 15 g sunflower oil
- 15 g balsamic vinegar
- 900 g Campbell's red and white vegetable beef soup bowl
- 2 thinly sliced green onion stalks
- 1 diced carrot
- 340 g cubed lean beef
- 1 Julienned celery stalk
- 1 Minced Garlic Clove
- 85 g pot barley

Directions:
1. Throw a cast iron pan or a deep saucepan on medium heat with the oil and cubed beef to allow the two to cook. Wait till beef is properly browned on all sides, and then add in the diced vegetables. Cover and cook for an additional 3-5 minutes, stirring occasionally.
2. Add in a combination of the broth, vinegar, and barley; reduce flame and bring to a boil. Continue to cook for about 20 minutes, or until thickened to preferred consistency.
3. Top with chopped green onions and serve!

Nutritional Information:
Calories: 279, Fat:7.6 g, Carbs:28.91 g, Protein:24.82 g, Sugars:3 g, Sodium:590 mg

Simple Pork and Capers

Prep time: 10 mins | Servings: 2

Ingredients:
- 8 oz. cubed pork
- 1 c. low-sodium chicken stock
- Black pepper
- 2 tbsps. Organic extra virgin olive oil
- 1 minced garlic oil
- 2 tbsps. Capers

Directions:

1. Heat up a pan with the oil over medium-high heat, add the pork season with black pepper and cook for 4 minutes on both sides.
2. Add garlic, capers and stock, stir and cook for 7 minutes more.
3. Divide everything between plates and serve.
4. Enjoy!

Nutritional Information:
Calories: 224, Fat:12 g, Carbs:12 g, Protein:10 g, Sugars:5 g, Sodium:5 mg

A "Boney" Pork Chop

Prep time: 20 mins | Servings: 4

Ingredients:
- 1 c. baby carrots
- Flavored vinegar
- 3 tbsps. Worcestershire sauce
- Ground pepper
- 1 chopped onion
- 4 ¾ bone-in thick pork chops
- ¼ c. divided butter
- 1 c. vegetables

Directions:
1. Take a bowl and add pork chops, season with pepper and flavored vinegar
2. Take a skillet and place it over medium heat, add 2 teaspoon of butter and melt it
3. Toss the pork chops and brown them
4. Each side should take about 3-5 minutes
5. Set your pot to sauté mode and add 2 tablespoon of butter, add carrots and sauté them
6. Pour broth and Worcestershire
7. Add pork chops and lock up the lid
8. Cook on HIGH pressure for 13 minutes
9. Release the pressure naturally
10. Enjoy!

Nutritional Information:
Calories: 715, Fat:37.4 g, Carbs:2 g, Protein:20.7 g, Sugars:0 g, Sodium:276 mg

Roast and Mushrooms

Prep time: 10 mins | Servings: 4

Ingredients:
- 1 tsp. Italian seasoning
- 12 oz. low-sodium beef stock
- 3 ½ lbs. pork roast
- 4 oz. sliced mushrooms

Directions:
1. In a roasting pan, combine the roast with mushrooms, stock and Italian seasoning, and toss
2. Introduce inside the oven and bake at 350 ^{0}F for starters hour and 20 minutes.
3. Slice the roast, divide it along while using mushroom mix between plates and serve.
4. Enjoy!

Nutritional Information:
Calories: 310, Fat:16 g, Carbs:10 g, Protein:22 g, Sugars:4 g, Sodium:600 mg

Easy Pork Chops

Prep time: 10 mins | Servings: 4

Ingredients:
- 1 c. low-sodium chicken stock
- 1 tsp. sweet paprika
- 4 boneless pork chops
- ¼ tsp. black pepper
- 1 tbsp. extra-virgin olive oil

Directions:
1. Heat up a pan while using the oil over medium-high heat, add pork chops, brown them for 5 minutes on either sides, add paprika, black pepper and stock, toss, cook for fifteen minutes more, divide between plates and serve by using a side salad.
2. Enjoy!

Nutritional Information:
Calories: 272, Fat:4 g, Carbs:14 g, Protein:17 g, Sugars:0.2 g, Sodium:68 mg

Pork and Celery Mix

Prep time: 10 mins | Servings: 8

Ingredients:
- 3 tsps. Fenugreek powder
- Black pepper
- 1 tbsp. organic olive oil
- 1 ½ c. coconut cream
- 26 oz. chopped celery leaves and stalks
- 1 lb. cubed pork meat
- 1 tbsp. chopped onion

Directions:
1. Heat up a pan while using oil over medium-high heat, add the pork as well as the onion, black pepper and fenugreek, toss and brown for 5 minutes.
2. Add the celery too because coconut cream, toss, cook over medium heat for twenty minutes, divide everything into bowls and serve.
3. Enjoy!

Nutritional Information:
Calories: 340, Fat:5 g, Carbs:8 g, Protein:14 g, Sugars:2.1 g, Sodium:200 mg

Pork and Dates Sauce

Prep time: ten mins | Servings: 6

Ingredients:
- 2 tbsps. Water
- 2 tbsps. Mustard
- 1/3 c. pitted dates
- Black pepper
- ¼ tsp. onion powder
- ¼ c. coconut aminos
- 1 ½ lbs. pork tenderloin
- ¼ tsp. smoked paprika

Directions:
1. In your blender, mix dates with water, coconut aminos, mustard, paprika, pepper and onion powder and blend well.
2. Put pork tenderloin within the roasting pan, add the dates sauce, toss to coat perfectly, introduce everything inside the oven at 400 °F, bake for 40 minutes, slice the meat, divide it as well since the sauce between plates and serve.
3. Enjoy!

Nutritional Information:
Calories: 240, Fat:8 g, Carbs:13 g, Protein:24 g, Sugars:0 g, Sodium:433 mg

Pork Roast and Cranberry Roast

Prep time: 10 mins | Servings: 4

Ingredients:
- 2 minced garlic cloves
- ½ tsp. grated ginger
- Black pepper
- ½ c. low-sodium veggie stock
- 1 ½ lbs. pork loin roast
- 1 tbsp. coconut flour
- ½ c. cranberries
- Juice of ½ lemon

Directions:
1. Put the stock in the little pan, get hot over medium-high heat, add black pepper, ginger, garlic, cranberries, fresh freshly squeezed lemon juice along using the flour, whisk well and cook for ten minutes.
2. Put the roast in the pan, add the cranberry sauce at the very top, introduce inside oven and bake at 375 °F first hour and 20 minutes.
3. Slice the roast, divide it along using the sauce between plates and serve.
4. Enjoy!

Nutritional Information:
Calories: 330, Fat:13 g, Carbs:13 g, Protein:25 g, Sugars:7 g, Sodium:150 mg

Pork and Roasted Tomatoes Mix

Prep time: 10 mins | Servings: 6

Ingredients:
- ½ c. chopped yellow onion
- 2 c. chopped zucchinis
- 1 lb. ground pork meat
- ¾ c. shredded low-fat cheddar cheese
- Black pepper
- 15 oz. no-salt-added, chopped and canned roasted tomatoes

Directions:
1. Heat up a pan over medium-high heat, add pork, onion, black pepper and zucchini, stir and cook for 7 minutes.
2. Add roasted tomatoes, stir, bring to a boil, cook over medium heat for 8 minutes, divide into bowls, sprinkle cheddar on the top and serve.
3. Enjoy!

Nutritional Information:
Calories: 270, Fat:5 g, Carbs:10 g, Protein:12 g, Sugars:8 g, Sodium:390 mg

Provence Pork Medallions

Prep time: 10 mins | Servings: 4

Ingredients:
- 1 tsp. Herb de Provence
- Pepper.
- ½ c. dry white wine
- 16 oz. pork tenderloins
- Salt

Directions:
1. Season pork lightly with salt and pepper.
2. Place the pork between two pieces of parchment paper and pound with a mallet.
3. You need to have ¼-inch thick meat.
4. In a large non-stick frying pan, cook the pork over medium-high heat for 2-3 minutes per side.
5. Remove from the heat and sprinkle with herb de Provence. Remove the pork from skillet and place aside. Keep warm.
6. Place the skillet over heat again. Add the wine and cook, stirring to scrape down the bits.
7. Cook until reduced slightly and pour over pork. Serve.

Nutritional Information:
Calories: 105.7, Fat:1.7 g, Carbs:0.8 g, Protein:22.6 g, Sugars:0 g, Sodium:67 mg

Garlic Pork Shoulder

Prep time: 10 mins | Servings: 6

Ingredients:
- 2 tsps. Sweet paprika
- 4 lbs. pork shoulder
- 3 tbsps. Extra virgin essential olive oil
- Black pepper
- 3 tbsps. Minced garlic

Directions:
1. In a bowl, mix extra virgin extra virgin olive oil with paprika, black pepper and oil and whisk well.
2. Brush pork shoulder with this mix, arrange inside a baking dish and introduce inside oven at 425 °F for twenty or so minutes.
3. Reduce heat to 325 °F F and bake for 4 hours.
4. Slice the meat, divide it between plates and serve having a side salad.
5. Enjoy!

Nutritional Information:
Calories: 321, Fat:6 g, Carbs:12 g, Protein:18 g, Sugars:0 g, Sodium:470 mg

Pork Patties

Prep time: 10 mins | Servings: 6

Ingredients:
- 10 oz. low sodium veggie stock
- ¼ c. no-salt-added tomato sauce
- 2 tbsps. Organic extra virgin olive oil
- ½ c. coconut flour
- ½ tsp. mustard powder
- Black pepper
- 1 ½ lbs. ground pork
- 2 whisked egg

Directions:
1. Put the flour in the very bowl too because egg in one more.
2. Mix the pork with black pepper also as a pinch of paprika, shape medium patties because of this mix, dip them inside egg then dredge in flour.
3. Heat up a pan while using oil over medium-high heat, add the patties and cook them for 5 minutes with them.
4. In a bowl, combine the stock with tomato sauce and mustard powder and whisk.
5. Add this over the patties, cook for ten minutes over medium heat, divide everything between plates and serve.
6. Enjoy!

Nutritional Information:
Calories: 332, Fat:18 g, Carbs:11 g, Protein:25 g, Sugars:0 g, Sodium:45 mg

Tarragon Pork Steak

Prep time: 10 mins | Servings: 4

Ingredients:
- 1 tbsps. Extra virgin olive oil
- Black pepper
- 4 medium pork steaks
- Chopped tarragon
- 8 halved cherry tomatoes

Directions:
1. Heat up a pan while using the oil over medium-high heat, add steaks, season with black pepper, cook them for 6 minutes on each side and divide between plates.
2. Heat the same pan over medium heat, add the tomatoes along with the tarragon, cook for ten minutes, divide next around the pork and serve.
3. Enjoy!

Nutritional Information:
Calories: 263, Fat:4 g, Carbs:12 g, Protein:16 g, Sugars:0.5 g, Sodium:762 mg

Pork Meatballs

Prep time: 10 mins | Servings: 4

Ingredients:
- 2 tbsps. Extra virgin olive oil
- 1 c. chopped red onion
- 1/3 c. chopped cilantro
- 4 minced garlic cloves
- 1 chopped Thai chili
- 1 lb. ground pork
- 1 tbsp. grated ginger

Directions:
1. In a bowl, combine the meat with cilantro, onion, garlic, ginger and chili, stir well and shape medium meatballs out of this mix.
2. Heat up a pan while using oil over medium-high heat, add the meatballs, cook them for 5 minutes on either side, divide them between plates and serve with a side salad.
3. Enjoy!

Nutritional Information:
Calories: 220, Fat:4 g, Carbs:8 g, Protein:14 g, Sugars:10 g, Sodium:592 mg

Winter Pork Roast

Prep time: 10 mins | Servings: 6

Ingredients:
- 1 tsp. powered cocoa
- 1 tsp. chili powder
- ½ tsp. onion powder
- 2 ½ lbs. pork roast
- Black pepper
- ¼ tsp. ground cumin

Directions:
1. In a roasting pan, combine the roast with black pepper, chili powder, onion powder, cumin and cocoa, rub, cover the pan, introduce inside oven and bake at 325 °F for 3 hours and twenty approximately minutes.
2. Slice, divide between plates and serve that features a side salad.
3. Enjoy!

Nutritional Information:
Calories:288 , Fat:5 g, Carbs:12 g, Protein:23 g, Sugars:0 g, Sodium:93 mg

Pork and Cabbage Salad

Prep time: 10 mins | Servings: 10

Ingredients:
- ½ c. low-fat sour cream
- 8 oz. drained and sliced water chestnuts
- 2 c. shredded already cooked pork roast
- 10 oz. peas
- ½ c. avocado mayonnaise
- 1 shredded green cabbage head
- 1 ½ c. already cooked brown rice
- ¼ tsp. black pepper

Directions:
1. In a bowl, combine the cabbage using the rice, shredded meat, peas, chestnuts, sour cream, mayo and black pepper, toss and serve cold.
2. Enjoy!

Nutritional Information:
Calories: 310, Fat:5 g, Carbs:11 g, Protein:17 g, Sugars:0 g, Sodium: 114 mg

Mustard Pork Chops

Prep time: 10 mins | Servings: 6

Ingredients:
- 1 tsp. sweet paprika
- Black pepper
- ½ tsp. dried oregano
- 2 pork chops
- 2 sliced yellow onions
- ¼ c. organic essential olive oil
- 2 tsps. Mustard
- 2 minced garlic cloves

Directions:
1. In a tiny bowl, mix oil with garlic, mustard, paprika, black pepper, and oregano and whisk well.
2. Add the pork chops, toss well leave aside to 10 minutes.
3. Place the meat for the preheated grill over medium-high heat and cook for 10 minutes on both sides.
4. Divide pork chops between plates and serve employing a side salad.
5. Enjoy!

Nutritional Information:
Calories: 314, Fat:4 g, Carbs:17 g, Protein:17 g, Sugars:0.04 g, Sodium:592 mg

Pork Chops and Apples

Prep time: 10 mins | Servings: 4

Ingredients:
- 1 chopped yellow onion
- 3 cored and sliced apples
- 1 ½ c. low-sodium chicken stock
- Black pepper
- 1 tbsp. extra virgin olive oil
- 4 pork chops
- 1 tbsp. chopped thyme

Directions:
1. Heat up a pan with all the oil over medium-high heat, add pork chops, season with black pepper and cook for 5 minutes on either side.
2. Add onion, garlic, apples, thyme and stock, toss, introduce inside oven and bake at 350 °F for 50 minutes.
3. Divide everything between plates and serve.
4. Enjoy!

Nutritional Information:
Calories: 340, Fat:12 g, Carbs:14 g, Protein:27 g, Sugars:0.2 g, Sodium:90 mg

Pork Belly and Apple Sauce

Prep time: 10 mins | Servings: 6

Ingredients:
- 2 lbs. trimmed and scored pork belly
- Virgin extra virgin olive oil
- 1 tbsp. freshly squeezed lemon juice
- 17 oz. cored and sliced apples
- Black pepper
- 2 c. low-sodium veggie stock
- 1 tsps. Sweet paprika

Directions:
1. In your blender, mix the stock with apples and lemon juice and pulse perfectly.
2. Put pork belly in a very roasting pan, add apple sauce, include the oil, paprika and black pepper, toss well, introduce inside oven and bake at 380 °F for one hour and half an hour.
3. Slice the pork belly, divide it between plates, drizzle the sauce across and serve.
4. Enjoy!

Nutritional Information:
Calories: 356, Fat:14 g, Carbs:10 g, Protein:27 g, Sugars:3 g, Sodium:333 mg

Pork and Fennel Mix

Prep time: 10 mins | Servings: 4

Ingredients:
- 4 halved figs
- 1/8 c. using apple cider vinegar
- 12 oz. cubed pork meat
- 2 tbsps. Extra virgin olive oil
- 2 sliced fennel bulbs
- Black pepper

Directions:
1. Heat up a pan with all the oil over medium-high heat, add the pork and brown for 5 minutes on both sides.
2. Add fennel, black pepper, figs and cider vinegar, toss, reduce heat to medium, cook for twenty or so minutes more, divide everything between plates and serve.
3. Enjoy!

Nutritional Information:
Calories: 260, Fat:3 g, Carbs:3.8 g, Protein:16 g, Sugars:0.1 g, Sodium:71 mg

Pork Chop Casserole

Prep time: 10 mins | Servings: 4

Ingredients:
- 1 finely crushed bay leaf
- ¾ c. lemon juice
- Chopped parsley
- 4 pork chops
- ¼ c. homemade chicken stock
- 1 thinly sliced onion
- 4 peeled and thinly sliced medium potatoes
- Black pepper

Directions:
1. Pour the oil in your pressure cooker and heat it.
2. Sprinkle the pork chops with pepper and salt and add to the pressure cooker. When the pork chops are seared, remove them and keep warm.
3. Use the chicken broth to deglaze the pressure cooker. This will loosen up the particles stuck to the bottom of the pressure cooker.
4. Add half of the onions and potatoes in the cooker and sprinkle with black pepper and chopped parsley.
5. Return the pork chops to the pressure cooker and sprinkle with the crushed bay leaf. Arrange the remaining potato and onion slices on top of the pork chops. Again, sprinkle with black pepper and chopped parsley.
6. Pour in the water and close and lock the lid. Cook on high pressure for 10 minutes. When the cooking time is up, release the pressure using the natural release method.

Nutritional Information:
Calories: 250, Fat:10 g, Carbs:15 g, Protein:16 g, Sugars:3 g, Sodium:508 mg

Pork and Red Peppers Mix

Prep time: 10 mins | Servings: 4

Ingredients:
- 1 tbsp. extra virgin essential olive oil
- ¼ c. low-sodium tomato sauce
- 2 chopped yellow onions
- 3 chopped red peppers
- Black pepper
- 1 ½ lbs. cubed pork meat
- 2 lbs. sliced Portobello mushrooms

Directions:
1. Heat up a pan with all the oil over medium-high heat, add the pork and brown it for 5 minutes.
2. Add sweet peppers, mushrooms and onions, stir and cook for 5 minutes more.
3. Add tomato sauce and black pepper, toss, introduce inside the oven and bake at 350 °F for 50 minutes.
4. Divide everything between plates and serve.
5. Enjoy!

Nutritional Information:
Calories: 130, Fat:12 g, Carbs:3 g, Protein:9 g, Sugars:2 g, Sodium:152 mg

Black Currant Jam Pork Chops

Prep time: 5 mins | Servings: 3

Ingredients:
- 3 orange slices
- Ground black pepper
- 1 tbsp. Dijon mustard
- 1/8 c. blackcurrant jam
- 8 oz. center cut pork loin chops
- 3 tbsps. Wine vinegar
- 1 tsp. olive oil

Directions:
1. Mix up the mustard and jam in a bowl. Set aside.

2. Heat olive oil in a nonstick skillet over medium-high heat.
3. Add the pork chops, cook for about five minutes on each side, until browned.
4. Place one tablespoon of the mustard/jam mixture on each pork chop. Cover the pan and cook for two minutes longer. Then, place the pork chops in plates.
5. Allow the skillet to cool to a warm temperature. Then, add the wine vinegar to the pan and stir to deglaze the browned bits.
6. Add the vinegar sauce to each plate of pork chop. Sprinkle black pepper on it and garnish with slices of orange.
7. Serve right away.

Nutritional Information:
Calories: 198, Fat:6 g, Carbs:11 g, Protein:25 g, Sugars:8 g, Sodium:188 mg

Pork and Cabbage Casserole

Prep time: 10 mins | Servings: 4

Ingredients:
- ½ c. coconut cream.
- 1 shredded green cabbage
- 1 tbsp. essential olive oil
- 2 minced garlic cloves
- Black pepper and salt
- 17 oz. cubed pork meat
- 1 chopped small yellow onion
- ½ c. grated low-fat parmesan

Directions:
1. Heat up a pot when using oil over medium-high heat, add onion, stir and cook for two main minutes.
2. Add garlic at the same time since the meat and brown for 5 minutes.
3. Add the cabbage, toss and cook everything for 10 minutes more.
4. Add black pepper and coconut cream and toss.
5. Sprinkle parmesan ahead, introduce the pan inside oven and bake at 350 °F for 20 minutes.
6. Enjoy!

Nutritional Information:
Calories: 260, Fat:7 g, Carbs:12 g, Protein:17 g, Sugars:3 g, Sodium:628 mg

Coconut Pork Chops

Prep time: 10 mins | Servings: 4

Ingredients:
- 4 pork chops
- 1 tbsp. chili powder
- 2 tbsps. olive oil
- 1 chopped yellow onion
- ¼ c. chopped cilantro
- 1 c. coconut milk

Directions:
1. Heat up a pan with the oil over medium-high heat, add the onion and the chili powder, toss and sauté for 5 minutes.
2. Add the pork chops and brown them for 2 minutes on each side.
3. Add the coconut milk, toss, bring to a simmer and cook over medium heat for 11 minutes more.
4. Add the cilantro, toss, divide everything into bowls and serve.

Nutritional Information:
Calories: 310, Fat:8 g, Carbs:16.7 g, Protein:22.1 g, Sugars:0.7 g, Sodium:303 mg

Curried Pork and Cabbage

Prep time: 10 mins | Servings: 4

Ingredients:
- 2 tbsps. Sliced green onion
- ¼ tsp. salt
- 2 tsps. Curry powder
- 32 oz. pork loin rib chops
- 4 c. shredded Napa cabbage
- 1 c. unsweetened pineapple juice

- ¼ tsp. ground black pepper
- 1 cored and sliced medium green cooking apple

Directions:
1. Trim fat from chops. Place chops in a 4- to 6-quart pressure cooker. In a small bowl, combine pineapple juice, curry powder, salt, and pepper; pour over meat.
2. Lock lid in place. Over high heat, bring cooker up to 15 pounds pressure. Reduce heat just enough to maintain high pressure. Cook for 3 minutes. Remove cooker from heat. Allow pressure to decrease naturally (this will take about 7 minutes).
3. Carefully remove the lid, tilting it away from you to allow steam to escape. Using a slotted spoon, transfer chops to a platter; cover to keep warm.
4. Bring the liquid in cooker to boiling. Add apple. Reduce heat. Simmer, uncovered, for 3 minutes, stirring occasionally.
5. Add Napa cabbage and green onion to cooker. Cook for 1 to 2 minutes more or until cabbage is wilted. Using a slotted spoon, transfer cabbage mixture to the platter with pork.
6. Transfer liquid in cooker to a small bowl or pitcher. To serve, pass liquid to spoon over chops and apple mixture.

Nutritional Information:
Calories: 102, Fat:4 g, Carbs:10 g, Protein:23 g, Sugars:07 g, Sodium:303 mg

Pork with Apple

Prep time: 15 mins | Servings: 8

Ingredients:
- 2 lbs. trimmed pork tenderloin
- 1 tsp. nutmeg
- 2 tbsps. Low-sodium soy sauce
- 4 cored and sliced apples

Directions:
1. Lightly, grease a slow cooker.
2. Place half of apple slice in the bottom of prepared slow cooker.
3. With a sharp knife, make slits into the pork.
4. Place the pork tenderloin over the apples slices. Sprinkle with half of nutmeg.
5. Place the remaining apple slices over pork tenderloin. Sprinkle with remaining nutmeg.
6. Pour soy sauce on top.
7. Set the slow cooker on low.
8. Cover and cook for about 6 hours.

Nutritional Information:
Calories: 311.5, Fat:18 g, Carbs:13.5 g, Protein:23.8 g, Sugars:0.2 g, Sodium:89 mg

Nutmeg Pork Chops

Prep time: 10 mins | Servings: 3

Ingredients:
- 1 chopped yellow onion
- 1 tbsp. balsamic vinegar
- ½ c. organic olive oil
- 3 boneless pork chops
- 8 oz. sliced mushrooms
- 2 tsps. Ground nutmeg
- ¼ c. coconut milk
- 1 tsp. garlic powder

Directions:
1. Heat up a pan using the oil over medium heat, add mushrooms and onions, stir and cook for 5 minutes.
2. Add pork chops, nutmeg and garlic powder and cook for 5 minutes more.
3. Add vinegar and coconut milk, toss, introduce inside oven and bake at 350 °F and bake for a half-hour.
4. Divide between plates and serve.
5. Enjoy!

Nutritional Information:
Calories: 260, Fat:10 g, Carbs:8 g, Protein:22 g, Sugars:2.4 g, Sodium:78 mg

Butter and Dill Pork Chops

Prep time: 5 mins | Servings: 4

Ingredients:
- ½ c. chicken broth
- ½ c. white wine
- 4 bone-in pork loin pieces
- 2 tbsps. unflavored vinegared butter
- 1 tbsp. minced fresh dill fronds
- ½ tsp. flavored vinegar
- ½ tsp. ground black pepper
- 16 baby carrots

Directions:
1. The first step here is to set your pot to sauté mode
2. Season the chops with pepper and flavored vinegar
3. Toss your chops into your pot and cook for 4 minutes
4. Transfer the chops to a plate and repeat to cook and brown the rest
5. Pour in 1 tablespoon of butter and Toss in your carrots, dill to the cooker and let it cook for about 1 minute
6. Pour in the wine and scrape off any browned bits in your cooker while the liquid comes to a boil
7. Stir in the broth
8. Return the chops to your pot
9. Lock up the lid and let it cook for about 18 minutes at high pressure
10. Naturally release the pressure by keeping it aside for 8 minutes
11. Unlock and serve with some sauce poured over

Nutritional Information:
Calories: 296, Fat:25 g, Carbs:0 g, Protein:17 g, Sugars:1.3 g, Sodium:155 mg

Paprika Pork with Carrots

Prep time: 10 mins | Servings: 4

Ingredients:
- 1 sliced red onion
- 1 lb. cubed pork stew meat
- 2 tbsps. olive oil
- ¼ c. low-sodium veggie stock
- Black pepper
- 2 peeled and sliced carrots
- 2 tsps. sweet paprika

Directions:
1. Heat up a pan with the oil over medium heat, add the onion, stir and sauté for 5 minutes.
2. Add the meat, toss and brown for 5 minutes more.
3. Add the rest of the ingredients, bring to a simmer and cook over medium heat for 20 minutes.
4. Divide the mix between plates and serve.

Nutritional Information:
Calories: 328, Fat:18.1 g, Carbs:6.4 g, Protein:34 g, Sugars:14 g, Sodium:399 mg

Pork and Greens Mix

Prep time: 10 mins | Servings: 4

Ingredients:
- 4 oz. mixed salad greens
- 1 tbsp. chopped chives
- 1/3 c. coconut aminos
- 2 tbsps. balsamic vinegar
- 1 tbsp. olive oil
- 4 oz. sliced pork stew meat
- 1 c. halved cherry tomatoes

Directions:
1. Heat up a pan with the oil over medium heat, add the pork, aminos and the vinegar, toss and cook for 15 minutes.
2. Add the salad greens and the other ingredients, toss, cook for 5 minutes more, divide between plates and serve.

Nutritional Information:
Calories: 125, Fat:6.4 g, Carbs:6.8 g, Protein:9.1 g, Sugars:0.2 g, Sodium:388.6 mg

Sage Pork Chops

Prep time: 10 mins | Servings: 4

Ingredients:
- 2 tbsps. olive oil
- 1 tbsp. lemon juice
- 4 pork chops
- 1 tbsp. chopped sage
- Black pepper
- 1 tsp. smoked paprika
- 2 minced garlic cloves

Directions:
1. In a baking dish, combine the pork chops with the oil and the other ingredients, toss, introduce in the oven and bake at 400 °F for 35 minutes.
2. Divide the pork chops between plates and serve with a side salad.

Nutritional Information:
Calories: 263, Fat:12.4 g, Carbs:22.2 g, Protein:16 g, Sugars:0 g, Sodium:960 mg

Pork with Avocados

Prep time: 10 mins | Servings: 4

Ingredients:
- 1 c. halved cherry tomatoes
- ½ c. low-sodium veggie stock
- 1 tbsp. olive oil
- 2 c. baby spinach
- 1 lb. sliced pork steak
- 2 peeled, pitted and sliced avocados
- 1 tbsp. balsamic vinegar

Directions:
1. Heat up a pan with the oil over medium-high heat, add the meat, toss and cook for 10 minutes.
2. Add the spinach and the other ingredients, toss, cook for 5 minutes more, divide into bowls and serve.

Nutritional Information:
Calories: 390, Fat:12.5 g, Carbs:16.8 g, Protein:13.5 g, Sugars:1 g, Sodium:0 mg

Pork with Chickpeas

Prep time: 10 mins | Servings: 4

Ingredients:
- 2 tbsps. chopped cilantro
- 1 lb. cubed pork stew meat
- Black pepper
- 10 oz. no-salt-added and chopped canned tomatoes
- 1 c. no-salt-added and drained canned chickpeas
- 1 tbsp. olive oil
- 1 chopped yellow onion

Directions:
1. Heat up a pan with the oil over medium-high heat, add the onion, toss and sauté for 5 minutes.
2. Add the meat, toss and cook for 5 minutes more.
3. Add the rest of the ingredients, toss, simmer over medium heat for 15 minutes, divide everything into bowls and serve.

Nutritional Information:
Calories: 476, Fat:17.6 g, Carbs:35.7 g, Protein:43.8 g, Sugars:6.8 g, Sodium:422.1 mg

Pork and Mint Corn

Prep time: 10 mins | Servings: 4

Ingredients:
- 1 c. corn
- 1 tbsp. chopped mint
- 1 c. low-sodium veggie stock
- Black pepper
- 1 tbsp. olive oil
- 1 tsps. sweet paprika
- 4 pork chops

Directions:
1. Put the pork chops in a roasting pan, add the rest of the ingredients, toss, introduce in the oven and bake at 380 °F for 1 hour.
2. Divide everything between plates and serve.

Nutritional Information:
Calories: 356, Fat:14 g, Carbs:11.0 g, Protein:1 g, Sugars:4.4 g, Sodium:349.5 mg

Pork Chops and Snow Peas

Prep time: 10 mins | Servings: 4

Ingredients:
- 2 tbsps. olive oil
- 1 c. low-sodium veggie stock
- 4 pork chops
- 1 c. snow peas
- 2 chopped shallots
- 1 tbsp. chopped parsley
- 2 tbsps. no-salt-added tomato paste

Directions:
1. Heat up a pan with the oil over medium heat, add the shallots, toss and sauté for 5 minutes.
2. Add the pork chops and brown for 2 minutes on each side.
3. Add the rest of the ingredients, bring to a simmer and cook over medium heat for 15 minutes.
4. Divide the mix between plates and serve.

Nutritional Information:
Calories: 357, Fat:27 g, Carbs:7.7 g, Protein:20.7 g, Sugars:5.3 g, Sodium:725.3 mg

Pork and Leeks Soup

Prep time: 10 mins | Servings: 4

Ingredients:
- 1 chopped yellow onion
- 6 c. low-sodium beef stock
- 5 chopped leeks
- 1 lb. cubed pork stew meat
- Black pepper
- 2 tbsps. olive oil
- 1 tbsp. chopped parsley

Directions:
1. Heat up a pot with the oil over medium-high heat, add the onion and the leeks, stir and sauté for 5 minutes.
2. Add the meat, stir and brown for 5 minutes more.
3. Add the rest of the ingredients, bring to a simmer and cook over medium heat for 30 minutes.
4. Ladle the soup into bowls and serve.

Nutritional Information:
Calories: 395, Fat:18.3 g, Carbs:18.4 g, Protein:38.2 g, Sugars:1 g, Sodium:770 mg

Pork with Peaches Mix

Prep time: 10 mins | Servings: 4

Ingredients:
- ¼ tsp. onion powder
- ¼ c. low-sodium veggie stock
- ¼ tsp. smoked paprika
- 2 lbs. roughly cubed pork tenderloin
- 2 tbsps. olive oil
- Black pepper
- 2 sliced peaches

Directions:
1. Heat up a pan with the oil over medium heat, add the meat, toss and cook for 10 minutes.
2. Add the peaches and the other ingredients, toss, bring to a simmer and cook over medium heat for 15 minutes more.
3. Divide the whole mix between plates and serve.

Nutritional Information:
Calories: 290, Fat:11.8 g, Carbs:13.7 g, Protein:24 g, Sugars:12 g, Sodium:628.9 mg

Allspice Pork Chops and Olives

Prep time: 10 mins | Servings: 4

Ingredients:
- 1 c. pitted and halved kalamata olives
- 1 chopped yellow onion
- 4 pork chops
- 2 tbsps. olive oil
- 1 tbsp. chopped chives
- ¼ c. coconut milk
- 1 tsp. ground allspice

Directions:
1. Heat up a pan with the oil over medium heat, add the onion and the meat and brown for 4 minutes on each side.
2. Add the rest of the ingredients, toss gently, introduce in the oven and bake at 390 °F for 25 minutes more.
3. Divide everything between plates and serve.

Nutritional Information:
Calories: 290, Fat:10 g, Carbs:7.8 g, Protein:22 g, Sugars:2 g, Sodium:821 mg

Pork Meatballs

Prep time: 10 mins | Servings: 4

Ingredients:
- 2 tbsps. avocado oil
- 1 tbsp. chopped cilantro
- 3 tbsps. almond flour
- 2 whisked egg
- 10 oz. no-salt-added canned tomato sauce
- Black pepper
- 2 lbs. ground pork

Directions:
1. In a bowl, combine the pork with the flour and the other ingredients except the sauce and the oil, stir well and shape medium meatballs out of this mix.
2. Heat up a pan with the oil over medium heat, add the meatballs and brown for 3 minutes on each side.
3. Add the sauce, toss gently, bring to a simmer and cook over medium heat for 20 minutes more.
4. Divide everything into bowls and serve.

Nutritional Information:
Calories: 332, Fat:18 g, Carbs:14.3 g, Protein:25 g, Sugars:0.14 g, Sodium:223 mg

Pork and Endives

Prep time: 10 mins | Servings: 4

Ingredients:
- 2 trimmed and shredded endives
- 1 chopped red onion
- 1 lb. cubed pork stew meat
- 1 c. low-sodium beef stock
- 1 tbsp. olive oil
- ¼ tsp. black pepper
- 1 tsp. chili powder

Directions:
1. Heat up a pan with the oil over medium heat, add the onion and the endives, toss and cook for 5 minutes.
2. Add the meat, toss and cook for 5 minutes more.
3. Add the rest of the ingredients, bring to a simmer and cook over medium heat for 25 minutes more.
4. Divide everything between plates and serve.

Nutritional Information:
Calories: 330, Fat:12.6 g, Carbs:10 g, Protein:22 g, Sugars:116 g, Sodium:0.1 mg

Pork with Brussels Sprouts

Prep time: 10 mins | Servings: 4

Ingredients:
- ½ lb. halved Brussels sprouts
- 1 tbsp. chopped cilantro
- Black pepper
- 2 lbs. cubed pork stew meat
- ¼ c. low-sodium tomato sauce
- 1 tbsp. olive oil
- 2 chopped spring onions

Directions:
1. Heat up a pan with the oil over medium-high heat, add the onions and the sprouts and brown for 5 minutes.
2. Add the meat and the other ingredients, bring to a simmer and cook over medium heat for 30 minutes more.
3. Divide everything between plates and serve.

Nutritional Information:
Calories: 541, Fat:25.6 g, Carbs:6.5 g, Protein:68.7 g, Sugars:3.2 g, Sodium:153 mg

Pork with Sprouts and Capers

Prep time: 10 mins | Servings: 4

Ingredients:
- 1 c. bean sprouts
- 1 c. low-sodium veggie stock
- 1 wedged yellow onion
- 2 tbsps. olive oil
- 1 lb. pork chops
- Black pepper
- 2 tbsps. drained capers

Directions:
1. Heat up a pan with the oil over medium-high heat, add the onion and the meat and brown for 5 minutes.
2. Add the rest of the ingredients, introduce the pan in the oven and bake at 390 °F for 30 minutes.
3. Divide everything between plates and serve.

Nutritional Information:
Calories: 324, Fat:12.5 g, Carbs:22.2 g, Protein:15.6 g, Sugars:0.1 g, Sodium:649 mg

Pork with Beets

Prep time: 10 mins | Servings: 4

Ingredients:
- 2 peeled and cubed small beets
- 1 chopped yellow onion
- 1 lb. cubed pork meat
- 2 minced garlic cloves
- 2 tbsps. olive oil
- Black pepper and salt
- ½ c. coconut cream.

Directions:
1. Heat up a pan with the oil over medium-high heat, add the onion and the garlic, stir and cook for 5 minutes.
2. Add the meat and brown for 5 minutes more.
3. Add the rest of the ingredients, bring to a simmer and cook over medium heat for 20 minutes.
4. Divide the mix between plates and serve.

Nutritional Information:
Calories: 331, Fat:14.3 g, Carbs:15.2 g, Protein:17 g, Sugars:18.5 g, Sodium:411.2 mg

Pork and Green Onions Mix

Prep time: 10 mins | Servings: 5

Ingredients:
- 1 tbsp. avocado oil
- 4 minced garlic cloves
- 1 lb. cubed pork meat
- 1 chopped green onion bunch
- Black pepper
- 1 c. low-sodium tomato sauce
- 1 chopped yellow onion

Directions:
1. Heat up a pan with the oil over medium-high heat, add the onion and green onions, stir and cook for 5 minutes.
2. Add the meat, stir and cook for 5 minutes more.
3. Add the rest of the ingredients, toss and cook over medium heat for 30 minutes more.
4. Divide everything into bowls and serve.

Nutritional Information:
Calories: 206, Fat:8.6 g, Carbs:7.2 g, Protein:23.4 g, Sugars:1 g, Sodium:1495 mg

Pork with Herbs de Provence

Prep time: 10 mins | Servings: 4

Ingredients:
- Freshly ground black pepper
- 8 oz. sliced pork tenderloin
- ¼ c. dry white wine
- ½ tsp. herbs de Provence

Directions:
1. Season pork pieces with black pepper and spread it between the wax paper.
2. Pound it with a mallet to get a ¼ inch thick pieces.
3. Heat a nonstick wok or frying pan and add pork to it.
4. Cook for 3 minutes per side until brown.
5. Drizzle herbs de Provence on top.
6. Transfer the pork to the serving plate.
7. Add wine to the same pan and cook until it boils.
8. Pour it over the pork and serve warm.

Nutritional Information:
Calories: 250, Fat:15.6 g, Carbs:1 g, Protein:23.6 g, Sugars:0.1 g, Sodium:482 mg

Pork and Carrots Soup

Prep time: 10 mins | Servings: 4

Ingredients:
- 1 lb. cubed pork stew meat
- 1 tbsp. chopped cilantro
- 1 tbsp. olive oil
- 1 chopped red onion
- 1 c. tomato puree
- 1 quart low-sodium beef stock
- 1 lb. sliced carrots

Directions:
1. Heat up a pot with the oil over medium-high heat, add the onion and the meat and brown for 5 minutes.
2. Add the rest of the ingredients except the cilantro, bring to a simmer, reduce heat to medium, and boil the soup for 20 minutes.
3. Ladle into bowls and serve for lunch with the cilantro sprinkled on top.

Nutritional Information:
Calories: 354, Fat:14.6 g, Carbs:19.3 g, Protein:36 g, Sugars:1 g, Sodium:354 mg

Chili Pork

Prep time: 10 mins | Servings: 4

Ingredients:
- 1 tbsp. chopped oregano
- 2 lbs. cubed pork stew meat
- 1 chopped yellow onion
- 2 tbsps. chili paste
- 2 minced garlic cloves
- 2 c. low-sodium beef stock
- 1 tbsp. olive oil

Directions:
1. Heat up a pot with the oil, over medium-high heat, add the onion and the garlic, stir and sauté for 5 minutes.
2. Add the meat and brown it for 5 minutes more.
3. Add the rest of the ingredients, bring to a simmer and cook over medium heat for 20 minutes more.
4. Divide the mix into bowls and serve.

Nutritional Information:
Calories: 363, Fat:8.6 g, Carbs:17.3 g, Protein:18.4 g, Sugars:2 g, Sodium:1127 mg

Chapter 7 Side Dishes and Appetizers

Cauliflower and Potato Mash

Prep time: 5 mins | Servings: 4

Ingredients:
- ½ tsp. flavored vinegar
- 1 minced garlic clove
- 2 lbs. Sliced potatoes
- 1 ½ c. water
- 8 oz. cauliflower florets

Directions:
1. Add water to your Instant Pot
2. Add potatoes and sprinkle cauliflower florets on top
3. Lock up the lid and cook on HIGH pressure for 5 minutes
4. Release the pressure naturally over 10 minutes
5. Sprinkle a bit of flavored vinegar and garlic
6. Mash and serve!

Nutritional Information:
Calories: 249, Fat:0.6 g, Carbs:55 g, Protein:7.5 g, Sugars:0.3 g, Sodium:56.3 mg

Grilled Asparagus

Prep time: 5 mins | Servings: 6

Ingredients:
- ¼ tsp. garlic powder
- 1 tbsp. olive oil
- ¼ tsp. salt
- 2 bunches trimmed asparagus
- 1 tsp. lemon zest

Directions:
1. Preheat the grill to 375 – 400F.
2. Add the trimmed asparagus spears to a baking sheet.
3. Drizzle the asparagus with olive oil, garlic powder and salt, and using clean hands toss the asparagus well to coat with the seasoning.
4. Place the asparagus directly onto the grill grates and grill for 3-4 minutes, until slightly caramelized.
5. Remove from the grill and season with the, fresh lemon zest, and serve.

Nutritional Information:
Calories: 45, Fat:2 g, Carbs:6 g, Protein:3 g, Sugars:1.2 g, Sodium:74 mg

Garlic Steamed Squash

Prep time: 5 mins | Servings: 4

Ingredients:
- 2 small zucchini
- Freshly ground black pepper
- All-purpose salt-free seasoning
- 2 medium yellow squash
- 6 peeled garlic cloves

Directions:
1. Trim the squash and zucchini and cut into 1-inch rounds.
2. Fill a steamer pot about 1 inch deep with water. Place pot over high heat and bring to a boil.
3. Place the veggies and garlic into the steamer basket. Place the steamer basket into the pot and cover tightly with lid. Steam for 10 minutes.
4. Remove pot from heat and carefully remove lid. Pluck garlic cloves from pot and gently mash with a fork.
5. Transfer the steamed veggies to a serving bowl, add the mashed garlic and toss gently to coat. Season to taste with all-purpose salt-free seasoning and freshly ground black pepper. Serve immediately.

Nutritional Information:
Calories: 38, Fat:0 g, Carbs:8 g, Protein:2 g, Sugars:2.1 g, Sodium:3.3 mg

Satisfying Corn Cob

Prep time: 5 mins | Servings: 8

Ingredients:
- 2 c. water
- 8 corn ears

Directions:
1. Husk the corns and cut the bottom part of the corns, wash them well thoroughly Wash well
2. Add water to the cooker base and arrange the corns vertically with the large part submerged underwater and the small part pointing upward
3. Lock up the lid and cook on HIGH pressure for 2 minutes
4. Release the pressure naturally
5. Serve with a bit of flavored vinegar and vegan butter

Nutritional Information:
Calories: 63, Fat:1 g, Carbs:14 g, Protein:2.4 g, Sugars:2.3 g, Sodium:2.5 mg

Devilled Eggs

Prep time: 10 mins | Servings: 12

Ingredients:
- 1/3 c. plain fat-free Greek yogurt
- ¼ tsp. ground black pepper
- 1 tsp. yellow mustard
- 1 tsp. white sugar
- 6 large eggs
- ¼ tsp. fine sea salt
- 1 tsp. red wine vinegar

Directions:
1. Put the eggs in a large, deep saucepan, and add enough water to completely cover them by ½ an inch.
2. Let the water boil, and then cook the eggs for 12 minutes.
3. Drain the hot water from the pan and cover the eggs in cold water. Rest the eggs rest for 2 minutes.
4. Drain the water and repeat this process until the eggs have completely cooled.
5. Peel the shell, and then halve each eggs lengthwise.
6. Separate the yolks from the whites.
7. Use only 5 of the 6 egg yolks, and put them in a small bowl.
8. Using a fork, mash the yolks until there are no large lumps, and then add the mustard, Greek yogurt, sugar, vinegar, salt, and pepper to the bowl. Stir this mixture until all the ingredients are well combined and smooth.
9. You may transfer this filling to a small plastic food storage bag, and snipping off one of the corners of the bag, make a piping bag or you may simply spoon the filling into the egg whites. .
10. Squeeze the egg yolk filling through hole in the piping bag into the egg whites, and serve garnish with paprika or parsley leaves, if desired.

Nutritional Information:
Calories: 37, Fat:2.1 g, Carbs:0.8 g, Protein:3.8 g, Sugars:0.33 g, Sodium:94 mg

Borders Apart Mexican Cauliflower Rice

Prep time: 5 mins | Servings: 4

Ingredients:
- 4 tbsps. Tomato paste
- 1 ½ c. water
- 1 can fire roasted tomatoes
- 3 c. chopped onion
- 6 c. cooked brown rice
- 2 c. salsa
- 6 garlic cloves

Directions:
1. Add the listed ingredients to your Instant Pot
2. Lock up the lid and cook on HIGH pressure for 5 minutes
3. Release the pressure naturally

4. Stir in chopped cilantro and top up with your desired toppings
5. Enjoy!

Nutritional Information:
Calories: 562, Fat:25 g, Carbs:63 g, Protein:23 g, Sugars:5.8 g, Sodium:201.2 mg

Egg and Bean Medley

Prep time: 5 mins | Servings: 3

Ingredients:
- 5 beaten eggs
- 1 tsp. chili powder
- 2 chopped garlic cloves
- ½ c. milk
- ½ c. tomato sauce
- 1 c. cooked white beans

Directions:
1. Add milk and eggs to a bowl and mix well
2. Add the rest of the ingredients and mix well
3. Add a cup of water to the pot
4. Transfer the bowl to your pot and lock up the lid
5. Cook on HIGH pressure for 18 minutes
6. Release the pressure naturally over 10 minutes
7. Serve with warm bread
8. Enjoy!

Nutritional Information:
Calories: 206, Fat:9 g, Carbs:23 g, Protein:9 g, Sugars:0.6 g, Sodium:917.2 mg

Cheddar and Apple Panini Sandwich

Prep time: 5 mins | Servings: 2

Ingredients:
- Cooking spray
- ½ c. arugula
- 4 whole-wheat bread slices
- 4 low-fat cheddar cheese slices
- 2 tbsps. low-fat honey mustard
- 1 thinly sliced apple

Directions:
1. Set Panini press on medium heat.
2. Spread the mustard on each slice of the bread. Lay the apple on two of the bread slices, top with cheese and then the arugula. Top with the other two slices of bread.
3. Coat the Panini press with cooking spray and grill each sandwich for 4-5 minutes.
4. Allow to cool before serving.

Nutritional Information:
Calories: 22, Fat:4 g, Carbs:23 g, Protein:11 g, Sugars:16 g, Sodium:570 mg

Roasted Carrots

Prep time: 15 mins | Servings: 4

Ingredients:
- 2 lbs. peeled and halved carrots
- ½ tsp. sea salt
- 2 tbsps. olive oil
- Flat leaf parsley
- 1 tbsp. raw honey
- ½ tsp. black pepper

Directions:
1. Preheat the oven to 400F.
2. Peel the carrots, cutting off the stems, and then cut the carrots in half creating a piece with a wide and narrow half.
3. Halve each carrot in half again lengthwise.
4. Place all the cut carrots into a bowl and add the olive oil, salt, pepper, and raw honey. Toss the carrots well to coat.
5. Spread the carrots evenly onto a baking sheet lined with aluminum foil, making sure they are all in a single layer.
6. Bake the carrots for 30 minutes, and then remove from oven to cool.
7. Garnish with fresh flat leaf parsley, if desired.

Nutritional Information:
Calories: 109, Fat:5.8 g, Carbs:14 g, Protein:1.4 g, Sugars:11 g, Sodium:264 mg

Fancy Red and White Sprouts

Prep time: 10 mins | Servings: 3

Ingredients:
- ¼ c. toasted pine nuts
- ½ tsp. flavored vinegar
- 1 grated pepper
- 1 lb. Brussels sprouts
- 1 pomegranate
- 1 tbsp. extra virgin olive oil

Directions:
1. Remove the outer leaves and trim the stems
2. Wash the Brussels
3. Cut the largest one in half and get all the ones in uniform size
4. Add 1 cup of water
5. Put steamer basket
6. Add sprouts to steamer basket
7. Lock up the lid and cook on HIGH pressure for 3 minutes
8. Release the pressure naturally
9. Move sprouts to serving dish and dress with olive oil, pepper and flavored vinegar
10. Sprinkle toasted pine nuts and pomegranate seeds
11. Serve and enjoy!

Nutritional Information:
Calories: 197, Fat:7 g, Carbs:22 g, Protein:6 g, Sugars:1.9 g, Sodium:22 mg

Garlic and Chive "Mash"

Prep time: 8 mins | Servings: 5

Ingredients:
- 2 lbs. peeled Yukon potatoes
- 4 peeled garlic cloves
- ¼ c. chopped chives
- ½ tsp. flavored vinegar
- 2 c. vegetable stock
- ½ c. almond milk

Directions:
1. Add broth, garlic and potatoes to the Instant Pot
2. Lock up the lid and cook on HIGH pressure for 9 minutes
3. Release the pressure naturally over 10 minutes
4. Drain just the amount of liquid required to maintain your required consistency
5. Mash the potatoes and stir in flavored vinegar and milk
6. Stir in chives and serve
7. Enjoy!

Nutritional Information:
Calories: 293, Fat:14 g, Carbs:35 g, Protein:8 g, Sugars:2.9 g, Sodium:313.7 mg

Crashing Asparagus Risotto with Microstock

Prep time: 10 mins | Servings: 2

Ingredients:
- 2 c. Arborio rice
- 1 medium size chopped red onion
- ½ tsp. lemon juice
- 4 c. water
- 1 lb. asparagus
- 2 tbsps. Olive oil
- ¼ c. white wine vinegar
- 2 tsps. Flavored vinegar

Directions:
1. Trim the asparagus by removing the stem, wash them under cold water and slice them in rondels making sure to keep the tips
2. Add woody stems and water to your Instant Pot
3. Lock up the lid and cook on HIGH pressure for 12 minutes, release the pressure naturally
4. Lift out the woody stem and discard the cooking liquid
5. Pour the liquid into a measuring cup
6. Add onion, olive oil to the pot and swirl

7. Add rice, onion and stir
8. Cook for 2 minutes
9. Splash in a bit of wine vinegar and deglaze
10. Add asparagus micro stock, asparagus rondels and tips
11. Season with flavored vinegar
12. Lock up the lid and cook on HIGH pressure for 6 minutes
13. Release the pressure naturally
14. Add a squeeze of lemon juice and serve
15. Enjoy!

Nutritional Information:
Calories: 486, Fat:7 g, Carbs:71 g, Protein:37 g, Sugars:0 g, Sodium:700.6 mg

Turkey and Melted Cheese Sandwich

Prep time: 10 mins | Servings: 2

Ingredients:
- 2 tsps. Dijon mustard
- ½ c. thinly sliced cucumber
- 2 whole-grain bread slices
- 2 low-sodium smoked turkey slices
- Pepper.
- ¼ c. shredded low-fat mozzarella

Directions:
1. Spread the mustard on each of the slices.
2. Lay the smoked turkey slice and then the cucumber slices on top of the bread. Sprinkle with the mozzarella and season with pepper.
3. Toaster to melt the cheese for about 3 minutes.
4. Serve while warm.

Nutritional Information:
Calories: 380, Fat:13.5 g, Carbs:40 g, Protein:25 g, Sugars:2.41 g, Sodium:550 mg

Garlic and Broccoli Mismash

Prep time: 3 mins | Servings: 4

Ingredients:
- 6 minced garlic cloves
- ½ c. water
- White wine vinegar
- Sea flavored vinegar
- 2 broccoli head cut up into florets
- 1 tbsp. peanut oil

Directions:
1. Place a steamer rack in your cooker
2. Add the florets to the rack
3. Add ½ a cup of water to the pot
4. Lock up the lid and cook on LOW pressure for 0 minutes
5. Quick release
6. Allow the broccoli to cool by transferring them to an ice bath
7. Remove water and set the pot to Sauté mode
8. Add 1 tablespoon of peanut oil alongside minced garlic
9. Sauté for 25-30 seconds and add the broccoli alongside 1 tablespoon of white wine vinegar
10. Season with a bit of flavored vinegar and stir for 30 seconds
11. Enjoy!

Nutritional Information:
Calories: 101, Fat:8 g, Carbs:6 g, Protein:6 g, Sugars:0.2 g, Sodium:41.5 mg

Crunchy Creamy Mashed Sweet Potatoes

Prep time: 5 mins | Servings: 4

Ingredients:
- ¼ tsp. nutmeg
- 1 c. water
- 2 lbs. Sliced garnet sweet potatoes
- Sea flavored vinegar
- 2 tbsps. Maple syrup
- 3 tbsps. Vegan butter

Directions:

1. Peel the sweet potatoes and cut up into 1 inch chunks
2. Pour 1 cup of water to the pot and add steamer basket
3. Add sweet potato chunks in the basket
4. Lock up the lid and cook on HIGH pressure for 8 minutes
5. Quick release the pressure
6. Open the lid and place the cooked sweet potatoes to the bowl
7. Use a masher to mash the potatoes
8. Add ¼ teaspoon of nutmeg, 2-3 tablespoon of unflavored vinegar butter, 2 tablespoon of maple syrup
9. Mash and mix
10. Season with flavored vinegar
11. Serve and enjoy!

Nutritional Information:
Calories: 249, Fat:8 g, Carbs:37 g, Protein:7 g, Sugars:13.9 g, Sodium:200 mg

Ultimate Roast Potatoes

Prep time: 5 mins | Servings: 4

Ingredients:
- Pepper
- 2 lbs. baby potatoes
- 3 skinned out garlic clove
- ½ c. stock
- 5 tbsps. Olive oil
- 1 rosemary sprig

Directions:
1. Set your pot to Sauté mode and add oil
2. Once it is heated up, add in the garlic, rosemary and potatoes
3. Sauté the potatoes for 10 minutes and brown them
4. Take a sharp knife and cut a small piece in the middle of your potatoes and pour the stock
5. Lock up the lid and cook on HIGH pressure for 7 minutes
6. Once done, wait for 10 minutes and release the pressure naturally
7. Add garlic cloves and peel the potatoes skin
8. Sprinkle a bit of pepper and enjoy!

Nutritional Information:
Calories: 42, Fat:1.3 g, Carbs:7.3 g, Protein:0.8 g, Sugars:1.7 g, Sodium:501 mg

Personal and Intimate Soy Milk

Prep time: 10 mins | Servings: 2

Ingredients:
- 5 c. water
- 1 vanilla bean extract piece
- ¼ tsp. cinnamon
- ½ c. organic yellow soy bean
- ½ tsp. stevia

Directions:
1. You need to soak the beans under water for about 36 hours prior to making the recipe
2. Strain the beans and replace old water with new after every 12 hours
3. Take a cutting board and chop up the soy beans
4. Take a small sized bowl and add the chopped up beans alongside ½ a cup of water
5. Add the mix to your blender and puree for 90 seconds
6. Pour the puree into your pot and add 5 cups of water
7. Give it a nice stir
8. Set your pot to Sauté mode and allow it to reach boiling point (foam will appear)
9. Stir it well and lock up the lid. Cook for 9 minutes under HIGH pressure
10. Allow the pressure to release naturally
11. Take another bowl and add stevia, vanilla bean extract, cinnamon and mix well
12. Open the lid and carefully strain the liquid into this bowl
13. Give it a nice stir and your milk is ready!
14. Enjoy

Nutritional Information:
Calories: 131, Fat:4.3 g, Carbs:15 g, Protein:23 g, Sugars:1 g, Sodium:81.9 mg

Extremely Crazy Egg Devils

Prep time: 5 mins | Servings: 6

Ingredients:
- Guacamole
- Furikake
- Mayonnaise
- 8 large eggs
- 1 c. water
- Sliced radishes

Directions:
1. Add 1 cup of water to your Instant Pot
2. Place the steamer insert in your pot
3. Arrange the eggs on top of the insert
4. Lock up the lid and cook for about 6 minutes at HIGH pressure
5. Allow the pressure to release naturally
6. Transfer the eggs to an ice bath and peel the skin
7. Cut the eggs in half and garnish them with dressings of Guacamole, sliced up radishes, Mayonnaise, Furikake, Sliced up Parmesan etc.!

Nutritional Information:
Calories: 137, Fat:10 g, Carbs:1 g, Protein:11 g, Sugars:1 g, Sodium:265 mg

Green Pea purée

Prep time: 20 mins | Servings: 2

Ingredients:
- 2 boiled sliced carrots
- ¼ c. 20% fat sour cream
- Pepper.
- 2 c. green peas
- Salt.

Directions:
1. Boil the carrots and the peas.
2. Using a blender purée the vegetables. Season with salt and pepper. Top with sour cream.

Nutritional Information:
Calories: 101, Fat:2.1 g, Carbs:14 g, Protein:7 g, Sugars:2.8 g, Sodium:57.2 mg

Herbed Green Beans

Prep time: 5 mins | Servings: 4

Ingredients:
- ½ c. chopped fresh mint
- 2 minced garlic cloves
- 1 tsp. lemon zest
- 4 c. trimmed green beans
- 1 tbsp. olive oil
- 1 tsp. coarse ground black pepper
- ½ c. chopped fresh parsley

Directions:
1. Heat the olive oil in a large sauté pan over medium heat. Add the green beans and garlic.
2. Sauté until the green beans are crisp tender, approximately 5-6 minutes.
3. Add the mint, parsley, lemon zest, and black pepper. Toss to coat.
4. Serve immediately.

Nutritional Information:
Calories: 66.2, Fat:3.5 g, Carbs:8.3 g, Protein:2.1 g, Sugars:2 g, Sodium:65 mg

Easy Lemon Roasted Radishes

Prep time: 5 mins | Servings: 2

Ingredients:
- 2 bunches rinsed and quartered radishes
- 2 tsps. Lemon juice
- Salt.
- 1½ tsp. roughly fresh chopped rosemary
- 1 tbsp. melted coconut oil
- Pepper

Directions:
1. Heat the oven to 350°F. Line a baking sheet with parchment paper.
2. Add pepper, salt, coconut oil, and radishes to a bowl and mix until combined.
3. Place the mixture on a baking sheet and bake for about 35 minutes, stirring occasionally.
4. When it is done, toss with rosemary and lemon juice.
5. Serve and enjoy.

Nutritional Information:
Calories: 37, Fat:2 g, Carbs:4 g, Protein:1 g, Sugars:2 g, Sodium:95 mg

Green Beans with Nuts

Prep time: 20 mins | Servings: 2

Ingredients:
- 3 minced garlic cloves
- 1 tbsp. olive oil
- ½ c. chopped walnuts
- 2 c. sliced green beans

Directions:
1. Boil the beans in salted water until tender.
2. Place the beans, garlic and walnuts in a preheated pan and cook for about 5-7 minutes on the stove.

Nutritional Information:
Calories: 285, Fat:24.1 g, Carbs:7.1 g, Protein:10 g, Sugars:3.3 g, Sodium:311 mg

Beets stewed with Apples

Prep time: 1 hour | Servings: 2

Ingredients:
- 2 tbsps. Tomato paste
- 1 tbsps. Olive oil
- 1 c. water
- 2 peeled, cored and sliced apples
- 3 peeled, boiled and grated beets
- 2 tbsps. Sour cream

Directions:
1. Boil the beets until half-done
2. In a deep pan preheated with olive oil cook the grated beets for 15 minutes.
3. Add the sliced apples, tomato paste, sour cream and 1 cup water. Stew for 30 minutes covered.

Nutritional Information:
Calories: 346, Fat:7.7 g, Carbs:26.8 g, Protein:2 g, Sugars:10.2 g, Sodium:96.1 mg

Cabbage Quiche

Prep time: 30 mins | Servings: 4

Ingredients:
- 2 beaten eggs
- 2 tbsps. Sour cream
- 2 tsps. Semolina
- Fresh parsley
- ½ shredded white cabbage head
- 2 tbsps. milk
- Salt

Directions:
1. In a saucepan stew the shredded cabbage with milk until soft and done.
2. Sprinkle the semolina over the cabbage, constantly stirring, and cook for 10 minutes more.
3. Remove from the heat, let cool and stir in the beaten eggs. Season with salt.
4. Arrange the cabbage mixture in a baking dish, coat with sour cream and bake at 400F for 20 minutes.
5. Serve with sour cream and fresh parsley leaves.

Nutritional Information:
Calories: 93, Fat:0.5 g, Carbs:27.8 g, Protein:19.4 g, Sugars:3.1 g, Sodium:561.6 mg

Baked Tomatoes

Prep time: 5 mins | Servings: 2

Ingredients:
- 2 minced garlic cloves
- 2 tbsps. Olive oil
- 2 sliced large tomatoes
- 2 tbsps. Minced basil
- 1 minced rosemary sprig

Directions:
1. Brush a baking sheet with olive oil.
2. Arrange the tomato slices on the baking sheet. Sprinkle with garlic, basil and rosemary. Brush with olive oil.
3. Bake in a preheated 350°F oven for 5-10 minutes.

Nutritional Information:
Calories: 161, Fat:14.5 g, Carbs:2 g, Protein:0.4 g, Sugars:2 g, Sodium:4 mg

Cabbage Rolls Stuffed with Dried Apricots

Prep time: 30 mins | Servings: 4

Ingredients:
- 4 tbsps. Rinsed and chopped dried apricots,
- 2 peeled, cored and grated apples
- 1/3 tsp. cinnamon
- 1 boiled cabbage head
- 2 tbsps. Rinsed raisins
- 1 tbsp. sugar

Directions:
1. Combine the grated apples, raisins, dried apricots, sugar and cinnamon.
2. Prepare the cabbage leaves: place the head of cabbage into water and bring to a boil. As the cabbage softens take it out, remove the outer leaves and carefully peel the leaves off one by one.
3. Spread the leaves out on paper towels and fill with apricot stuffing. Roll them up.
4. Place the rolls into preheated to 400F oven for 40 minutes.

Nutritional Information:
Calories: 175, Fat:0.4 g, Carbs:16.6 g, Protein:10.8 g, Sugars:2.9 g, Sodium:980.4 mg

Rice and Chicken Stuffed Tomatoes

Prep time: 10 mins | Servings: 4

Ingredients:
- 1 pack grilled and sliced chicken breast
- 2 tbsps. Chopped basil leaf
- 2 c. cooked brown rice
- 1 tbsp. olive oil
- 4 large tomatoes
- ½ c. grated parmesan cheese
- 2 minced garlic cloves

Directions:
1. Set the oven at 350F.
2. Take the top of the tomatoes off and then carefully scoop the seeds using a spoon.
3. In a large bowl, mix together the cooked brown rice, chicken, basil, garlic, and parmesan (leave about 1 tsp. of parmesan). Use this mixture to stuff the tomatoes.
4. Sprinkle the stuffed tomatoes with the remaining parmesan. Place them in an oven-safe dish and brush with the olive oil.
5. Place in the oven to cook for 25 minutes.
6. Let it cool down before serving.

Nutritional Information:
Calories: 230, Fat:4.1 g, Carbs:27.3 g, Protein:21.5 g, Sugars:2.9 g, Sodium:407.7 mg

Squash Pancakes

Prep time: 10 mins | Servings: 4

Ingredients:
- 2 beaten eggs
- Salt
- Sour cream
- 2 peeled, deseeded and grated medium summer squashes
- 1 tbsp. flour

Directions:
1. Drain the liquid from the grated squashes.
2. Add eggs, flour and season with salt. Mix well. Form this mixture into pancakes.
3. Line a baking sheet with parchment paper and scoop the pancakes onto it.
4. Bake in the oven at 400F for 20-30 minutes.
5. Serve with sour cream.

Nutritional Information:
Calories: 31, Fat:0.4 g, Carbs:12.7 g, Protein:5.8 g, Sugars:3.4 g, Sodium:41.7 mg

Avocado Dip

Prep time: 5 mins | Servings: 2

Ingredients:
- ½ c. low-fat sour cream
- 2 tsps. minced onions
- 1/8 tsp. hot sauce
- 1 peeled, pitted and mashed avocado

Directions:
1. Mix all the ingredients together in a blender and blend until smooth.
2. Serve with tortilla chips.

Nutritional Information:
Calories: 217, Fat:17.3 g, Carbs:7 g, Protein:1.6 g, Sugars:0.6 g, Sodium:44.5 mg

Stuffed Turnips

Prep time: 5 mins | Servings: 4

Ingredients:
- 2 peeled and grated carrots
- 2 tbsps. Olive oil
- 2 tbsps. Honey
- 4 rinsed turnips.
- 2 peeled and grated apples

Directions:
1. Preheat the oven to 400°F.
2. Mix grated carrots with grated apples in honey.
3. Boil the turnips until half-done.
4. When the turnips are cool enough to handle, cut off the tops and scoop out some of the flesh.
5. Rub the turnips inside with olive oil and fill with vegetable stuffing.
6. Bake for 1 hr.

Nutritional Information:
Calories: 197, Fat:7.3 g, Carbs:8 g, Protein:4 g, Sugars:3.5 g, Sodium:61.3 mg

Apples Stuffed with Quark

Prep time: 5 mins | Servings: 4

Ingredients:
- 8 oz. cottage cheese
- 1 tsp. confectioners' sugar
- 2 tbsps. Sugar
- 4 cored apples
- 1 whisked egg
- 1 tbsp. raisins

Directions:
1. Combine the quark with egg, sugar and raisins. Mix well.

2. Scrape out the some of the apples' flesh and fill with quark mixture.
3. Place on a baking sheet and bake at 400F for 20 minutes.

Nutritional Information:
Calories: 189, Fat:0.6 g, Carbs:9 g, Protein:12 g, Sugars:20 g, Sodium:108 mg

Baked Pumpkin Oatmeal

Prep time: 30 mins | Servings: 4

Ingredients:
- 3¼ c. water
- 2 tbsps. Sour cream
- 1 c. peeled, cored and grated pumpkin
- 2 tbsps. Sugar
- 2 c. oats
- 1 c. milk
- 2 egg whites

Directions:
1. In a medium saucepan prepare the oatmeal: bring 3¼ cups water to a boil and stir in the oats. Add sugar. Stir constantly until thick.
2. In a skillet add ½ cup milk, grated pumpkin and simmer until the pumpkin is half-cooked.
3. Combine oatmeal with pumpkin.
4. Whisk the egg whites until smooth. Add to pumpkin-oatmeal mixture.
5. Pour the mixture into a baking pan and bake at 400F for 30 minutes.
6. Serve with sour cream.

Nutritional Information:
Calories: 189, Fat:3.1 g, Carbs:57 g, Protein:6.3 g, Sugars:14.2 g, Sodium:224.2 mg

Meringue Cookies

Prep time: 5 mins | Servings: 4

Ingredients:
- 2 tbsps. Sugar
- 3 beaten egg whites

Directions:
1. Using a blender beat the cooled egg whites on high.
2. Constantly blending add sugar little by little.
3. Line a baking sheet with parchment paper. Using an icing bag, squeeze our portions of the egg mixture unto the parchment paper.
4. Place into a preheated to 155°F oven for 15 min.

Nutritional Information:
Calories: 35, Fat:0 g, Carbs:6 g, Protein:0.4 g, Sugars:6 g, Sodium:10.7 mg

Rose Hip Jelly

Prep time: 7 hours | Servings: 2

Ingredients:
- 2 c. water
- 1 tsp. gelatin
- 2 tbsps. Sugar
- 2 tbsps. Rinsed and crushed rose-hip berries
- 2 lemon slices

Directions:
1. Bring the 2 cups water to a boil, add the crushed rose hips and boil for 5 minutes.
2. Leave the hips in the liquid to infuse for 6 hours. Then strain the infusion through a sieve, retaining the liquid.
3. Dissolve sugar in ½ cup of rose-hip water and bring to boil. Add the remaining rose-hip water and lemon slices.
4. Soak the gelatin in cool water for 25-30 minutes.
5. Add the gelatin to the rose-hip extract and bring to a boil. Take it from the heat immediately and pour into molds or jars.
6. Place in the fridge to cool and thicken.

Nutritional Information:
Calories: 45, Fat:0 g, Carbs:11 g, Protein:0 g, Sugars:2.6 g, Sodium:4 mg

Easy Broccoli and Penne

Prep time: 10 mins | Servings: 3

Ingredients:
- 3 chopped garlic cloves
- 6 oz. uncooked whole-wheat penne
- Ground pepper
- 3 c. roughly chopped broccoli florets
- 1 tbsp. olive oil
- 2 tbsps. Grated Romano cheese

Directions:
1. Cook the penne in a pot according to the package instructions. Add the florets to cook with the pasta.
2. Before draining, take ¼ cup of the pasta water and set aside.
3. Place the pot back to the stove and heat the olive oil over high heat. Sauté the garlic for about a minute.
4. Reduce the heat and then add the pasta and broccoli to the pot. Stir well.
5. Add the Romano and ¼ cup of the pasta water. Mix well. Season with pepper.

Nutritional Information:
Calories: 419.8, Fat:12.9 g, Carbs:52 g, Protein:32.2 g, Sugars:2.4 g, Sodium:540.5 mg

Berry Soufflé

Prep time: 15 mins | Servings: 2

Ingredients:
- 2 tbsps. sugar
- ½ c. water
- 3 oz. rinsed berries
- 3 egg whites

Directions:
1. Combine the berries sugar and water in a saucepan and boil until thick.
2. Using an electric beater beat the egg whites until foamy.
3. Constantly stirring, combine the berry mixture with egg whites.
4. Pour the soufflé mixture into a mold.
5. Bake at 390°F for 15 minutes.
6. Serve immediately, sprinkled with confectioners' sugar if desired.

Nutritional Information:
Calories: 79, Fat:0.4 g, Carbs:28.6 g, Protein:8.3 g, Sugars:8.3 g, Sodium:36.7 mg

White Sponge Cake

Prep time: 15 mins | Servings: 4

Ingredients:
- 1 tbsp. sugar
- 1 tbsp. flour
- 2 egg whites

Directions:
1. Using an electric mixer beat the egg whites until foamy.
2. Slowly add sugar, continuing to whisk.
3. Slowly add the flour, constantly stirring.
4. Pour the mixture into a silicone mold.
5. Bake at 400F for 20 min. Check for doneness with a toothpick.

Nutritional Information:
Calories: 23, Fat:0.1 g, Carbs:36.4 g, Protein:4.6 g, Sugars:46 g, Sodium:144 mg

Roasted Asparagus

Prep time: 1 hour | Servings: 2

Ingredients:
- Black pepper
- 1 tsp. olive oil
- 2 c. quartered mushrooms
- Zest of 1 lemon
- 1 lb. sliced asparagus
- 2 tbsps. Balsamic vinegar

Directions:
1. In a bowl combine all ingredients until well coated.
2. Place into the fridge for 1 hour to marinate.
3. Broil the asparagus mixture under high heat until lightly browned.

Nutritional Information:
Calories: 143, Fat:7.6 g, Carbs:3.9 g, Protein:22 g, Sugars:1.2 g, Sodium:74 mg

Rigatoni with Broccoli

Prep time: 5 mins | Servings: 2

Ingredients:
- 3 minced garlic cloves
- 2 tbsps. grated parmesan cheese
- Pepper.
- 1/3 lb. rigatoni pasta
- 2 c. broccoli florets
- 2 tsps. olive oil

Directions:
1. Fill a large saucepan with water and bring to a boil. Following the instructions on the package add the pasta and cook until al dente.
2. In a separate pot add 1 inch water and bring to boil. Put the broccoli florets into a steamer basket and steam for 10 minutes.
3. In a large bowl combine the cooked pasta with broccoli. Toss with garlic, olive oil, Parmesan cheese, and black pepper.

Nutritional Information:
Calories: 46.2, Fat:14.9 g, Carbs:25 g, Protein:14 g, Sugars:2 g, Sodium:640 mg

Rutabaga Puree

Prep time: 10 mins | Servings: 4

Ingredients:
- 2 c. low sodium vegetable broth
- 1 tbsp. fresh tarragon
- 4 c. chopped rutabaga
- 2 tsps. fresh thyme
- 2 c. unsweetened coconut milk
- ½ c. low-fat sour cream

Directions:
1. In a large saucepan, bring the coconut milk and vegetable broth to a boil.
2. Add the rutabaga, reduce heat, and let simmer for 30 minutes.
3. Remove from heat and strain the rutabaga, reserving the liquid.
4. Using a blender or immersion blender, blend until smooth, adding the reserved liquid as desired to reach preferred consistency.
5. Season with tarragon and thyme.
6. Serve immediately.

Nutritional Information:
Calories: 207.2, Fat:16.7 g, Carbs:11.8 g, Protein:3.4 g, Sugars:10.8 g, Sodium:39 mg

Pan Seared Acorn Squash and Pecans

Prep time: 5 mins | Servings: 6

Ingredients:
- 1 tsp. chopped rosemary
- 1 c. sliced sweet yellow onion
- 2 tbsps. vegetable oil
- 4 c. cubed acorn squash
- 1 tbsp. honey
- 1 c. chopped pecans

Directions:
1. Add the vegetable oil to a sauté pan over medium high heat.
2. Add the onion and sauté until tender, 2-3 minutes.
3. Add the acorn squash, tossing gently for 5-7 minutes.
4. Add the honey, pecans, and rosemary. Stir to coat and cook an additional 3 minutes.
5. Serve warm.

Nutritional Information:
Calories: 222.3, Fat:17.6 g, Carbs:17.4 g, Protein:2.7 g, Sugars:0.9 g, Sodium:92.5 mg

Shaved Brussels Sprouts with Walnuts

Prep time: 10 mins | Servings: 4

Ingredients:
- ½ c. fresh shaved parmesan
- 1 tsp. thyme
- 2 tbsps. olive oil
- 1 tsp. black pepper
- ½ c. chopped walnuts
- ½ c. diced red onion
- 4 c. shaved Brussels sprouts

Directions:
1. Heat the olive oil in a skillet over medium heat. Add the onions and sauté until tender, approximately 2-3 minutes.
2. Add the Brussels sprouts and cook for 5 minutes. Season with thyme and black pepper.
3. Remove from heat and stir in the walnuts.
4. Garnish with fresh Parmesan for serving.

Nutritional Information:
Calories: 173.0, Fat:12.8 g, Carbs:10.0 g, Protein:5.7 g, Sugars:2.7 g, Sodium:220 mg

Honey Mustard Chicken Fillets

Prep time: 10 mins | Servings: 4

Ingredients:
- ¼ c. Dijon mustard
- 3 tsps. raw honey
- 4 packs chicken fillets
- ½ juice of lime
- ¼ c. toasted slivered almonds
- 1 minced garlic clove

Directions:
1. Pre-heat grill to medium-high heat.
2. In a small bowl, combine the Dijon mustard, honey and lime juice. Whisk well.
3. Using this mixture, brush the chicken fillets on each side.
4. When the grill is hot, cook the chicken fillets for 12-15 minutes turning and brushing with the sauce occasionally.
5. Garnish with the toasted slivered almonds on top before serving.

Nutritional Information:
Calories: 192.7, Fat:2.5 g, Carbs:10.2 g, Protein:27.3 g, Sugars:8.6 g, Sodium:122.1 mg

Grilled Pesto Shrimps

Prep time: 10 mins | Servings: 2

Ingredients:
- Kosher salt
- 1 garlic clove
- ¼ kg. peeled and deveined large shrimp
- ½ c. chopped basil
- Ground pepper
- Skewers
- 2 tbsps. olive oil
- 2 tbsps. parmesan cheese

Directions:
1. Place the fresh basil, garlic, cheese, salt and pepper in a food processor and pulse. Gradually add the oil to the mixture until you create a pesto sauce.
2. Place the shrimps in a bowl and pour over the pesto sauce. Toss gently and let it marinate in t fridge for at least an hour.
3. When you're ready to cook, pre-heat your grill to medium-low heat.
4. Thread the shrimps into the skewers and cook on the grill for about 3-4 minutes on each side.
5. Serve warm with a bowl of yogurt and fresh fruits.

Nutritional Information:
Calories: 219.7, Fat:7.8 g, Carbs:22.2 g, Protein:15.1 g, Sugars:1.7 g, Sodium:238.7 mg

Rosemary Potato Shells

Prep time: 5 mins | Servings: 2

Ingredients:
- Butter-flavored cooking spray
- 2 medium russet potatoes
- 1/8 tsp. freshly ground black pepper
- 1 tbsp. minced fresh rosemary

Directions:
1. Switch on the oven and set it to 375 °F to preheat.
2. Pierce the mashed potatoes with a fork and place them in a baking sheet.
3. Bake for 1 hour until crispy.
4. Allow the potatoes to cool for handling then cut them in half.
5. Scoop out the pulp leaving the 1/8-inch-thick shell.
6. Brush the shells with melted butter and season with pepper and rosemary.
7. Bake for another 5 minutes.
8. Serve.

Nutritional Information:
Calories: 167, Fat:0 g, Carbs:27 g, Protein:7.6 g, Sugars:1.5 g, Sodium:200.7 mg

Basil Tomato Crostini

Prep time: 10 mins | Servings: 4

Ingredients:
- ¼ c. minced fresh basil
- ¼ lb. sliced and toasted Italian bread
- 4 chopped plum tomatoes
- 2 tsps. olive oil
- Freshly ground pepper
- 1 minced garlic clove

Directions:
1. Toss tomatoes with oil, garlic, pepper, and basil in a bowl.
2. Cover and allow them sit for 30 minutes.
3. Top the toasts with this mixture.
4. Serve.

Nutritional Information:
Calories: 104, Fat:3.5 g, Carbs:15 g, Protein:3 g, Sugars:0.3 g, Sodium:7.5 mg

Cranberry Spritzer

Prep time: 10 mins | Servings: 4

Ingredients:
- 1 c. raspberry sherbet
- 1-quart sugar-free cranberry juice
- ¼ c. sugar
- 10 lemon wedges
- ½ c. fresh lemon juice
- 1-quart carbonated water

Directions:
1. Refrigerate carbonated water, lemon juice, and cranberry juice until cold.
2. Mix cranberry juice with sugar, sherbet, lemon juice, and carbonated water.
3. Garnish with a lemon wedge.
4. Serve.

Nutritional Information:
Calories: 50, Fat:0 g, Carbs:15.1 g, Protein:1.2 g, Sugars:45 g, Sodium:65 mg

Butternut Squash Fries

Prep time: 10 mins | Servings: 4

Ingredients:
- 1 tbsp. olive oil
- 1 tbsp. chopped fresh thyme
- 1 medium butternut squash
- ½ tsp. salt
- 1 tbsp. chopped fresh rosemary

Directions:
1. Switch on the oven and set it to 425 °F to preheat.
2. Layer a baking sheet with cooking spray.
3. Peel the squash and slice into 3-inch-long and ½ inch wide.
4. Place the pieces in a large bowl and toss with oil, thyme, salt, and rosemary.
5. Spread the squash in the baking sheet and bake for 10 minutes.
6. Toss the fries well and bake again for 5 minutes or more until golden brown.
7. Serve.

Nutritional Information:
Calories: 62, Fat:2 g, Carbs:11 g, Protein:11 g, Sugars:5 g, Sodium:164.1 mg

Chapter 8 Snacks and Desserts

Healthy Chocolate Avocado Pudding

Prep time: 2 mins | Servings: 2

Ingredients:
- 6 tbsps. unsweetened coconut milk
- Crushed almonds
- 2 tbsps. raw honey
- Toasted coconut flakes
- 1 ripe avocado
- ¼ tsp. sea salt
- 3 tbsps. cocoa powder

Directions:
1. Add all the ingredients for the pudding to a food processor or high-speed blender.
2. Blend thoroughly until smooth and chill for about 15 minutes.
3. When ready to serve, top with the crushed almonds and toasted coconut flakes.
4. Enjoy.

Nutritional Information:
Calories: 123, Fat:9.4 g, Carbs:20.9 g, Protein:2.5 g, Sugars:1.4 g, Sodium:18.6 mg

Date-a-Peanut Snack Bars

Prep Time: 15 mins | Servings: 10

Ingredients:
- 420 g roasted peanuts
- 2 ½ g. salt
- 30 pitted dates

Directions:
1. Go ahead and throw your dates all into the food processor and add the salt and blend until it forms a smooth paste.
2. Add in the roasted peanuts and pulse until the nuts are coarsely chopped and grab a spoon and make a big ball of date-nut dough.
3. Roll your dough into a 1 inch thick mat and cut into sticks or bars and serve.

Nutritional Information:
Calories: 307, Fat:21 g, Carbs:25 g, Protein:11 g, Sugars:8 g, Sodium:150 mg

Lemony Chickpeas Dip

Prep time: 10 mins | Servings: 4

Ingredients:
- ½ c. chopped coriander
- Zest one grated lemon
- 1 tbsp. olive oil
- 4 tbsps. pine nuts
- Juice of one lemon
- 14 oz. no-salt-added drained and rinsed canned chickpeas

Directions:
1. In a blender, combine the chickpeas with lemon zest, freshly squeezed lemon juice, coriander and oil, pulse well, divide into small bowls, sprinkle pine nuts at the pinnacle and serve as a conference dip.
2. Enjoy!

Nutritional Information:
Calories: 200, Fat:12 g, Carbs:9 g, Protein:7 g, Sugars:1 g, Sodium:350 mg

Baked Stuffed Apples

Prep time: 10 mins | Servings: 3-4

Ingredients:
- ½ c. orange juice
- ¼ c. flaked coconut
- 2 tsps. grated orange zest
- 2 tbsps. brown sugar
- 4 Golden delicious apples
- ¼ c. chopped dried apricots

Directions:
1. Dress off the one-third of the apple and clear the middle with the help of a knife. Organize the fruit on a plate which is microwave proof.
2. Mix coconut, orange zest and apricots and level it to put it in the middle of the apple.
3. Combine orange juice and brown sugar, and put it over apples. Use a plastic to cover the lid and the microwave on high for 7 to 8 minutes till it is tender.
4. Serve it cool.

Nutritional Information:
Calories: 359.4, Fat:2.2 g, Carbs:10.6 g, Protein:1.5 g, Sugars:22 g, Sodium:48.9 mg

Basmati Rice Pudding with Oranges

Prep time: 15 mins | Servings: 3-4

Ingredients:
- 3 large navel oranges
- ¼ c. low-fat sweetened condensed milk
- 4 tbsps. sugar
- ¾ c. Basmati rice white rice
- ½ halved vanilla bean
- 4 c. fat-free evaporated milk

Directions:
1. Take a 2 quart pan and boil 2 cups of water, add rice and cover it with lowering the heat.
2. Cook it for 20 minutes till it is soft and the water is taken up by the rice. Take a clean orange, extract 1 teaspoon of zest from it.
3. Cut it in half and juice it, save it. Remove the rind from rest of the oranges, extract the white pith. Clear the bifurcations.
4. When the rice is soft, add half cup of the orange juice, the zest, evaporated milk, condensed milk, vanilla bean and sugar.
5. Cook the mix over medium flame for 20 to 25 minutes, without the cover, stirring regularly till it creams up.
6. Clear off the vanilla bean and pour the rice mixture among bowls to serve hot.

Nutritional Information:
Calories: 230.5, Fat:6.7 g, Carbs:39 g, Protein:4.2 g, Sugars:28.2 g, Sodium:51.3 mg

Berry Yogurt Popsicles

Prep time: 30 mins | Servings: 2-3

Ingredients:
- 1 c. blackberries
- 1 ¼ c. non-fat milk
- 1 c. non-fat plain yogurt
- 1 c. blueberries

Directions:
1. Put all the material in a blender and put in half cup of smoothie mix upon your cups and put in the freezer for half an hour.
2. Take it out and put in the sticks and put them back in for an hour or so.

Nutritional Information:
Calories: 44, Fat:0.8 g, Carbs:8 g, Protein:2 g, Sugars:28 g, Sodium:7 mg

Chili Nuts

Prep time: 10 mins | Servings: 4

Ingredients:
- 14 oz. mixed nuts
- ½ tsp. ginger powder
- 1 egg white
- ½ tsp. curry powder
- 4 tbsps. coconut sugar
- ½ tsp. chili flakes
- ¼ tsp. cayenne

Directions:
1. In a bowl, combine the egg white with all the chili flakes, curry powder, curry powder, ginger powder, coconut sugar and cayenne and whisk well.
2. Add the nuts, toss well, spread them having a lined baking sheet, introduce within the oven and bake at 400 °F for ten minutes.
3. Divide the nuts into bowls and serve as a snack.
4. Enjoy!

Nutritional Information:
Calories: 234, Fat:12 g, Carbs:14 g, Protein:7 g, Sugars:5 g, Sodium:1000 mg

Apples and Cream Shake

Prep time: 10 mins | Servings: 3-4

Ingredients:
- 1 c. unsweetened applesauce
- ¼ tsp. ground cinnamon
- 1 c. fat-free skim milk
- 2 c. vanilla low-fat ice cream

Directions:
1. Use a blender to mix low-fat ice cream, applesauce and cinnamon and blend it with the lid on.
2. Put in add fat free milk skim and cover again and till it mixes up.
3. After this pour and serve instantly.

Nutritional Information:
Calories: 269.4, Fat:10.5 g, Carbs:37.6 g, Protein:8.6 g, Sugars:31.2 g, Sodium:106.2 mg

Lemony Kale Popcorn

Prep time: 5 mins | Servings: 4

Ingredients:
- 2 tsps. grape seed oil
- 2 tsps. lemon zest
- 10 c. popped popcorn
- ¼ tsp. sea salt
- ½ bunch chopped kale

Directions:
1. Preheat the oven to 325F.
2. Pat the kale completely dry with kitchen paper and then coat with olive oil and salt.
3. Place onto the baking sheet and bake for 11 minutes until crispy.
4. Stir once or twice halfway through cooking and be careful that the kale does not burn.
5. Remove the kale and let cool.
6. Place the cooled kale into a food processor together with the lemon zest and process into a fine powder.
7. Add this seasoning to the prepared popcorn and serve.

Nutritional Information:
Calories: 131, Fat:4 g, Carbs:22 g, Protein:5 g, Sugars:0 g, Sodium:250 mg

Perfect Hard-Boiled Eggs

Prep time: 5 mins | Servings: 8

Ingredients:
- 8 whole eggs
- 5 g salt
- 85 g white vinegar
- 2 liters water
- 5 g black pepper

Directions:
1. Put your water, vinegar and spices in a saucepan and allow the water to come to a slow boil.
2. Add all 8 eggs carefully into the water and turn down the heat and cook for about 15 minutes.
3. Once done, pour the water out and run the eggs under cold or iced water, to prevent overcooking.
4. Cool, peel and eat!

Nutritional Information:
Calories: 56, Fat:4.5 g, Carbs:1 g, Protein:3 g, Sugars:0.6 g, Sodium:63 mg

Chickpeas and Pepper Hummus

Prep time: 10 mins | Servings: 4

Ingredients:
- Juice of ½ lemon
- 4 chopped walnuts
- 1 tbsp. sesame paste
- 14 oz. no-salt-added, drained and rinsed canned chickpeas
- 2 chopped roasted red peppers

Directions:
1. In your blender, combine the chickpeas with all the sesame paste, red peppers, lemon juice and walnuts, pulse well, divide into bowls and serve as being a snack.
2. Enjoy!

Nutritional Information:
Calories: 231, Fat:12 g, Carbs:15 g, Protein:14 g, Sugars:0.2 g, Sodium:412.2 mg

Tortilla Chips

Prep time: 10 mins | Servings: 6

Ingredients:
- ¼ tsp. cayenne
- 2 tbsps. organic extra virgin olive oil
- 12 whole wheat grain tortillas
- 1 tbsp. chili powder

Directions:
1. Spread the tortillas for the lined baking sheet, add the oil, chili powder and cayenne, toss, introduce inside oven and bake at 350 °F for 25 minutes.
2. Divide into bowls and serve as a side dish.
3. Enjoy!

Nutritional Information:
Calories: 199, Fat:3 g, Carbs:12 g, Protein:5 g, Sugars:0 g, Sodium:9.8 mg

Almond Rice Pudding

Prep time: 10 mins | Servings: 3-4

Ingredients:
- ¼ c. sugar
- 1 tsp. vanilla
- 3 c. milk
- 1 c. white rice
- ¼ c. toasted almonds
- Cinnamon
- ¼ tsp. almond extract

Directions:
1. Get the milk and rice together in a pan and boil and simmer it by lowering the heat for

half an hour with the top on till the rice softens up a bit.
2. Take it off the burner and put in sugar, almond, vanilla and cinnamon.
3. Garish roasted almonds at the top and eat it warm.

Nutritional Information:
Calories: 80, Fat:1.5 g, Carbs:16 g, Protein:1 g, Sugars:7 g, Sodium:121.4 mg

Sweet Potatoes and Apples Mix

Prep time: 10 mins | Servings: 1

Ingredients:
- 1 tbsp. low-fat butter
- ½ lb. cored and chopped apples
- 2 tbsps. water
- 2 lbs. sweet potatoes

Directions:
1. Arrange the potatoes around the lined baking sheet, bake inside oven at 400 °F for an hour, peel them and mash them in the meat processor.
2. Put apples in the very pot, add the river, bring using a boil over medium heat, reduce temperature, and cook for ten minutes.
3. Transfer to your bowl, add mashed potatoes, stir well and serve every day.
4. Enjoy!

Nutritional Information:
Calories: 140, Fat:1 g, Carbs:8 g, Protein:6 g, Sugars:2.6 g, Sodium:493.3 mg

Sautéed Bananas with Orange Sauce

Prep time: 5 mins | Servings: 4

Ingredients:
- ¼ c. frozen pure orange juice concentrate
- 2 tbsps. margarine
- ¼ c. sliced almonds
- 1 tsp. orange zest
- 1 tsp. fresh grated ginger
- 4 firm, sliced ripe bananas
- 1 tsp. cinnamon

Directions:
1. Melt the margarine over medium heat in a large skillet, until it bubbles but before it begins to brown.
2. Add the cinnamon, ginger, and orange zest. Cook, while stirring, for 1 minute before adding the orange juice concentrate. Cook, while stirring until an even sauce has formed.
3. Add the bananas and cook, stirring carefully for 1-2 minutes, or until warmed and evenly coated with the sauce.
4. Serve warm with sliced almonds.

Nutritional Information:
Calories: 164.3, Fat:9.0 g, Carbs:21.4 g, Protein:2.3 g, Sugars:26 g, Sodium:100 mg

Caramelized Blood Oranges with Ginger Cream

Prep time: 10 mins | Servings: 4

Ingredients:
- 2 tbsps. low sugar orange marmalade
- 1 tbsp. divided fresh grated ginger
- 4 c. peeled and sliced blood oranges
- 2 tbsps. brown sugar
- Candied orange peel
- ½ c. coconut cream

Directions:
1. Begin by preheating the broiler.
2. In a small saucepan combine the orange marmalade and two teaspoons of the fresh ginger. Heat over low heat and stir until the mixture becomes slightly liquefied.
3. Place a thin layer of the oranges into the bottom of four large baking ramekins and then brush with the marmalade mixture. Repeat this step until all of the oranges have been used. Pour any remaining gingered marmalade over the tops of the ramekins.

4. Sprinkle each ramekin with brown sugar and place under the broiler for approximately 5 minutes, or until caramelized.
5. Serve warm garnished with coconut cream and candied orange peel, if desired.
6. To make the coconut cream: Take one can of pure, unsweetened coconut milk and place it in your refrigerator for 24 hours. Take the can out of the refrigerator and scoop out the thick cream that has settled on top. Place this in a bowl, along with one teaspoon of ginger and beat until creamy.

Nutritional Information:
Calories: 220.2, Fat:10.7 g, Carbs:32.4 g, Protein:2.4 g, Sugars:19.5 g, Sodium:143.7 mg

Grilled Minted Watermelon

Prep time: 10 mins | Servings: 4

Ingredients:
- 1 tbsp. honey
- ¼ c. finely chopped fresh mint
- 8 thick deseeded watermelon slices

Directions:
1. Prepare and preheat a stovetop grill.
2. Lightly press towels against the watermelon slices to remove as much excess moisture as possible.
3. Lightly brush both sides of the watermelon slices with honey.
4. Place the watermelon slices on the grill and grill for approximately 3 minutes per side, or until slightly caramelized.
5. Serve warm, sprinkled with fresh mint.

Nutritional Information:
Calories: 199.2., Fat:2.6 g, Carbs:45.7 g, Protein:3.8 g, Sugars:10.4 g, Sodium:219.8 mg

Caramelized Apricot Pots

Prep time: 10 mins | Servings: 6

Ingredients:
- ¼ c. white sugar
- 2 tsps. lemon juice
- ½ tsp. thyme
- 3 c. sliced apricots
- 1 tbsp. brown sugar
- 1 c. part skim ricotta cheese
- 1 tsp. lemon zest

Directions:
1. Preheat the broiler of your oven.
2. Place the apricots in a bowl and toss with the lemon juice.
3. In another bowl, combine the ricotta cheese, thyme, and lemon zest. Mix well.
4. Spread a layer of the ricotta mixture into the bottoms of 6 large baking ramekins.
5. Spoon the apricots over the top of the ricotta cheese in each.
6. Combine the white sugar and brown sugar. Sprinkle evenly over the apricots, avoiding large clumps of sugar as much as possible.
7. Place the ramekins under the broiler for approximately 5 minutes, or until caramelized.
8. Serve warm.

Nutritional Information:
Calories: 133.6, Fat:3.6 g, Carbs:21.6 g, Protein:5.8 g, Sugars:6 g, Sodium:206 mg

Melon Mojito Granita

Prep time: 10 mins | Servings: 6

Ingredients:
- ¼ c. chopped fresh mint
- ¼ c. lime juice
- 4 c. cubed cantaloupe melon
- 1 c. peach nectar

Directions:
1. Combine the melon, peach nectar, lime juice, and mint in a blender or food processor. Blend until smooth.

2. Place the mixture in a shallow metal pan and place in the freezer.
3. Check the mixture every 30 minutes or so. Using a spoon or fork, mix and scrape the mixture at every check, until a slushy ice has formed. This will take a couple of hours.
4. Take out of the freezer and let soften slightly before serving.
5. Serve with fresh fruit, if desired.

Nutritional Information:
Calories: 55.7, Fat:0 g, Carbs:13.8 g, Protein:0.8 g, Sugars:12.5 g, Sodium:3 mg

Mocha Pops

Prep Time: 10 mins | Servings: 4-6

Ingredients:
- ½ tsp. pure vanilla extract
- 2 tbsps. honey
- ½ c. chopped almonds
- ¼ c. cooled brewed espresso
- 2 c. coconut milk
- 2 tbsps. dark cocoa powder

Directions:
1. In a blender, combine the coconut milk, honey, cocoa powder, espresso, and vanilla extract. Blend until creamy.
2. Pour the mixture into freeze pop molds and sprinkle with almonds.
3. Place in the freezer and freeze for at least 4 hours before enjoying.

Nutritional Information:
Calories: 317.3, Fat:27.3 g, Carbs:17.3 g, Protein:4.6 g, Sugars:5 g, Sodium:26 mg

Rhubarb Pie

Prep time: 10 mins | Servings: 12

Ingredients:
- 4 c. chopped rhubarb
- 8 oz. low-fat cream cheese
- 1 c. melted low-fat butter
- 1 ¼ c. coconut sugar
- 2 c. whole wheat flour
- 1 c. chopped pecans
- 1 c. sliced strawberries

Directions:
1. In a bowl, combine the flour while using the butter, pecans and ¼ cup sugar and stir well.
2. Transfer this for some pie pan, press well in for the pan, introduce inside the oven and bake at 350 °F for 20 minutes.
3. In a pan, combine the strawberries with all the current rhubarb, cream cheese and 1 cup sugar, stir well and cook over medium heat for 4 minutes.
4. Spread this inside the pie crust whilst inside fridge for the couple hours before slicing and serving.
5. Enjoy!

Nutritional Information:
Calories: 162, Fat:5 g, Carbs:15 g, Protein:6 g, Sugars:16.6 g, Sodium:411 mg

Berry No Bake Bars

Prep time: 10 minutes | Servings: 18

Ingredients:
- 1 c. natural peanut butter
- ¼ c. chopped dried blueberries
- 3 c. oatmeal
- ¼ c. chopped dried cranberries
- 3 tbsps. honey

Directions:
1. Line a baking pan with wax paper or parchment paper.

2. Microwave the peanut butter for 10-15 seconds, just until it softens and begins to liquefy.
3. Combine the oatmeal, peanut butter, honey, cranberries, and blueberries together in a bowl and mix until blended.
4. Spread the mixture out evenly into the pan.
5. Place in the refrigerator and let set for 2 hours before cutting into squares.

Nutritional Information:
Calories: 145.0, Fat:6.4 g, Carbs:17.9 g, Protein:4.4 g, Sugars:17.9 g, Sodium:102.4 mg

Tropical Fruit Napoleon

Prep time: 20 mins | Servings: 6-8

Ingredients:
- 1 tbsp. finely chopped fresh lemongrass
- 1 c. cubed mango
- 1 tsp. vanilla extract
- 1 peeled and cored whole pineapple
- 1 c. shredded unsweetened coconut
- 2 c. cubed papaya
- 2 c. light whipping cream

Directions:
1. Add the vanilla extract to the whipping cream and beat until thick and creamy. Fold in the coconut and lemongrass. Place in the refrigerator to chill for at least 30 minutes.
2. Cut the pineapple in thin, lengthwise pieces, creating "sheets" of pineapple.
3. Mix the mango and papaya together in a bowl.
4. Lay one-third of the pineapple sheets on a work surface
5. Spread a third of the whipping cream onto the pineapple.
6. Top with some mango and papaya. Follow this with another layer of pineapple, cream, and fruit.
7. Top with a final layer of pineapple, cream, and fruit.
8. Serve chilled and garnish with additional lemongrass, if desired.

Nutritional Information:
Calories: 128.5, Fat:6.9 g, Carbs:17.7 g, Protein:1.0 g, Sugars:6 g, Sodium:80 mg

Ginger Peach Pie

Prep time: 10 mins | Servings: 10

Ingredients:
- 5 c. diced peaches
- ½ c. sugar
- 2 refrigerated whole wheat pie crust doughs
- 1 tsp. cinnamon
- ½ c. orange juice
- ¼ c. chopped candied ginger
- ½ c. cornstarch

Directions:
1. Preheat the oven to 425°F.
2. Place one of the pie crusts in a standard size pie dish. Spread some coffee beans or dried beans in the bottom of the pie crust to use as a weight. Place the dish in the oven and bake for 10-15 minutes, or until lightly golden. Remove from the oven and let cool.
3. Combine the peaches, candied ginger, and cinnamon in a bowl. Toss to mix.
4. Combine the sugar, cornstarch, and orange juice in a saucepan and heat over medium until syrup begins to thicken.
5. Pour the syrup over the peaches and toss to coat.
6. Spread the peaches in the pie crust and top with the remaining crust. Crimp along the edges and cut several small slits in the top.
7. Place in the oven and bake for 25-30 minutes, or until golden brown.
8. Let set before slicing.

Nutritional Information:
Calories: 289.0, Fat:13.1 g, Carbs:41.6 g, Protein:3.9 g, Sugars:22 g, Sodium:154 mg

Mocha Ricotta Cream

Prep time: 10 mins | Servings: 4

Ingredients:
- 2 c. part skin ricotta cheese
- 1 tbsp. espresso powder
- Almond cookie crumbs
- ½ c. powdered sugar
- 1 tbsp. dark cocoa powder
- 1 tsp. pure vanilla extract

Directions:
1. Combine the ricotta cheese, powdered sugar, espresso powder, cocoa powder, and vanilla extract in a bowl.
2. Using an electric mixer, blend until creamy.
3. Cover and refrigerate for at least 4 hours.
4. Serve in individual dishes, garnished with cookie crumbs, if desired.

Nutritional Information:
Calories: 230.6, Fat:9.9 g, Carbs:22.0 g, Protein:14.3 g, Sugars:3.2 g, Sodium:166 mg

Fresh Parfait

Prep time: 10 mins | Servings: 6

Ingredients:
- 4 peeled and chopped grapefruits
- 2 tsps. grated lime zest
- 4 c. non-fat yogurt
- 2 tbsps. lime juice
- 1 tbsp. chopped mint
- 3 tbsps. stevia

Directions:
1. In a bowl, combine the yogurt using the stevia, lime juice, lime zest and mint and stir.
2. Divide the grapefruits into small cups, add the yogurt mix in each and serve.
3. Enjoy!

Nutritional Information:
Calories: 200, Fat:3 g, Carbs:15 g, Protein:10 g, Sugars:20 g, Sodium:13 mg,

Easy Fudge

Prep time: 2-3 hours | Servings: 12

Ingredients:
- ½ c. low-fat butter
- 2 c. coconut sugar
- 1 c. non-fat milk
- 1 tsp. vanilla flavoring
- 12 oz. chopped chocolate brown

Directions:
1. Heat up a pan while using milk over medium heat, add the sugar as well as the butter, stir and cook everything for 7 minutes.
2. Take this off heat, add the chocolate and whisk everything.
3. Pour this right into a lined square pan, spread well, keep within the fridge for two main hours, cut into small squares and serve.
4. Enjoy!

Nutritional Information:
Calories: 154, Fat:5 g, Carbs:16 g, Protein:3 g, Sugars:16 g, Sodium:10 mg

Fruit Skewers

Prep time: 10 mins | Servings: 10

Ingredients:
- 1 cored and sliced apple
- ¼ cubed cantaloupe
- 5 halved strawberries
- 2 sliced bananas

Directions:

1. Thread strawberry, cantaloupe, bananas and apple chunks alternately onto skewers and serve them cold.
2. Enjoy!

Nutritional Information:
Calories: 76, Fat:1 g, Carbs:10 g, Protein:2 g, Sugars:9 g, Sodium:6 mg

Easy Pomegranate Mix

Prep time: 10 mins | Servings: 2

Ingredients:
- Single pomegranate seeds
- 2 c. pomegranate juice
- 1 c. steel cut oats

Directions:
1. In a bit pot, combine the pomegranate juice with pomegranate seeds and oats, toss, cook over medium heat for 5 minutes, divide into bowls and serve cold.
2. Enjoy!

Nutritional Information:
Calories: 172, Fat:4 g, Carbs:10 g, Protein:5 g, Sugars:24 g, Sodium:5 mg

Berries Mix

Prep time: 10 mins | Servings: 6

Ingredients:
- 4 tbsps. coconut sugar
- 2 tsps. freshly squeezed fresh lemon juice
- 1 lb. strawberries
- 1 lb. blackberries

Directions:
1. In a pan, combine the strawberries with blackberries and sugar, stir, provide your simmer over medium heat and cook for ten minutes.
2. Divide into cups and serve cold.
3. Enjoy!

Nutritional Information:
Calories: 120, Fat:2 g, Carbs:4 g, Protein:4 g, Sugars:9 g, Sodium:2 mg,

Broccoli Bites

Prep time: 5 mins | Servings: 4

Ingredients:
- 80 g olive oil
- 10 g garlic chili infused oil
- 1 ½ lbs. chopped broccoli
- 2 g ground black pepper
- 4 minced garlic cloves
- 2 g salt

Directions:
1. Preheat oven to about 400 ºF.
2. In a large bowl, add the chopped broccoli, spices and olive oil, and toss until well-seasoned. Put the broccoli in a baking sheet and bake for about 15-20 minutes.
3. Pull out and drizzle with infused oils, before baking for an additional 5 minutes.
4. Pull out and serve, fresh!

Nutritional Information:
Calories: 94, Fat:6.4 g, Carbs:7 g, Protein:6 g, Sugars:11 g, Sodium:389 mg

Coconut Mousse

Prep time: 10 mins | Servings: 12

Ingredients:
- 1 tsp. vanilla flavoring
- 1 tsp. coconut extract
- 1 c. toasted coconut
- 2 ¾ c. coconut milk
- 4 tsps. coconut sugar

Directions:

1. In a bowl, combine the coconut milk with the coconut extract, vanilla flavor, coconut and sugar, whisk well, divide into small cups and serve cold.
2. Enjoy!

Nutritional Information:
Calories: 152, Fat:5 g, Carbs:11 g, Protein:3 g, Sugars:0.1 g, Sodium:13 mg

Blueberry Cream

Prep time: 5 mins | Servings: 1

Ingredients:
- 1 tbsp. low-fat peanut butter
- 2 dates
- ¾ c. blueberries
- 1 peeled banana
- ¾ c. almond milk

Directions:
1. In a blender, combine the blueberries with peanut butter, milk, banana and dates, pulse well, divide into small cups and serve cold.
2. Enjoy!

Nutritional Information:
Calories: 120, Fat:3 g, Carbs:6 g, Protein:7 g, Sugars:2.5 g, Sodium:55 mg

Lemon Apple Mix

Prep time: 10 mins | Servings: 6

Ingredients:
- 4 tbsps. coconut sugar
- 2 tsps. vanilla flavoring
- 2 tsps. cinnamon powder
- 2 tsps. lemon juice
- 6 cored and chopped apples

Directions:
1. In a little pan, combine the apples with all the sugar, vanilla, fresh lemon juice and cinnamon, toss, heat over medium heat, cook for 10-15 minutes, divide between small dessert plates and serve.
2. Enjoy!

Nutritional Information:
Calories: 120, Fat:4 g, Carbs:8 g, Protein:5 g, Sugars:13 g, Sodium:175 mg

Minty Rhubarb

Prep time: 10 mins | Servings: 4

Ingredients:
- 1/3 c. water
- 2 lbs. roughly chopped rhubarb
- 1 tbsp. chopped mint
- 3 tbsps. coconut sugar

Directions:
1. Put the river inside a tiny pot, get hot over medium heat, add the sugar and whisk well.
2. Add rhubarb and mix, toss, cook for 10 minutes, divide into bowls and serve.
3. Enjoy!

Nutritional Information:
Calories: 160, Fat:2 g, Carbs:8 g, Protein:5 g, Sugars:15 g, Sodium:39 mg

Nigella Mango Sweet Mix

Prep time: 10 mins | Servings: 8

Ingredients:
- 1 tsp. cinnamon powder
- 1 ½ lbs. peeled and cubed mango
- 3 tbsps. coconut sugar
- ½ c. apple cider vinegar treatment
- 1 tsp. nigella seeds

Directions:

1. In a tiny pot, combine the mango while using nigella seeds, sugar, vinegar and cinnamon, toss, bring using a simmer over medium heat, cook for 10 minutes, divide into bowls and serve.
2. Enjoy!

Nutritional Information:
Calories: 160, Fat:3 g, Carbs:8 g, Protein:3 g, Sugars:6 g, Sodium:147 mg

Blueberry Compote

Prep time: 10 mins | Servings: 6

Ingredients:
- 1 lb. blueberries
- 1 oz. orange juice
- 5 tbsps. coconut sugar

Directions:
1. In a pot, combine the sugar with all the orange juice and blueberries, toss, bring which has a boil over medium heat, cook for 15 minutes, divide into bowls and serve cold.
2. Enjoy!

Nutritional Information:
Calories: 120, Fat:2 g, Carbs:6 g, Protein:9 g, Sugars:3 g, Sodium:1 mg

Lentils and Dates Brownies

Prep time: 10 mins | Servings: 8

Ingredients:
- 1 peeled and chopped banana
- 2 tbsps. powered cocoa
- ½ tsp. baking soda
- 28 oz. no-salt-added, rinsed and drained canned lentils
- 1 tbsp. coconut sugar
- 4 tbsps. almond butter
- 12 dates

Directions:
1. Put lentils inside food processor, pulse, add dates, sugar, banana, baking soda, almond butter and cocoa powder, pulse well, pour right in to a lined pan, spread, bake inside oven at 375°F for quarter-hour, leave the amalgamation aside to cool down the down a little bit, cut into medium pieces and serve.
2. Enjoy!

Nutritional Information:
Calories: 202, Fat:4 g, Carbs:12 g, Protein:6 g, Sugars:8 g, Sodium:8 mg

Blueberry Curd

Prep time: 10 mins | Servings: 4

Ingredients:
- 12 oz. blueberries
- 3 tbsps. coconut sugar
- 2 eggs
- 2 tbsps. melted coconut oil
- 2 tbsps. fresh lemon juice

Directions:
1. Put the oil in a pot, get hot over medium heat, add freshly squeezed freshly squeezed lemon juice and coconut sugar and whisk well.
2. Add the blueberries plus the eggs, whisk well, cook for ten minutes, divide into small cups and serve cold.
3. Enjoy!

Nutritional Information:
Calories: 201, Fat:3 g, Carbs:6 g, Protein:3 g, Sugars:8 g, Sodium:10 mg

Almond Peach Mix

Prep time: 10 mins | Servings: 4

Ingredients:
- 2 c. rolled oats
- ½ c. chopped almonds
- 1 chopped peach
- 4 c. water
- 2 tbsps. flax meal
- 1 tsp. vanilla flavoring

Directions:
1. In a pan, combine water while using oats, vanilla flavoring, flax meal, almonds and peach, stir, give a simmer over medium heat, cook for 10 minutes, divide into bowls and serve.
2. Enjoy!

Nutritional Information:
Calories: 161, Fat:3 g, Carbs:7 g, Protein:5 g, Sugars:8.5 g, Sodium:17.5 mg

Coconut Cream

Prep time: 1 hour | Servings: 4

Ingredients:
- 1 tsp. cinnamon powder
- 5 tbsps. coconut sugar
- 2 c. coconut cream
- Zest of one grated lemon
- 3 whisked eggs

Directions:
1. In just a little pan, combine the cream with cinnamon, eggs, sugar and lemon zest. Whisk well
2. Simmer over medium heat for 10 minutes.
3. Divide into ramekins and inside fridge for an hour before serving.
4. Enjoy!

Nutritional Information:
Calories: 130, Fat:5 g, Carbs:8 g, Protein:6 g, Sugars:1.8 g, Sodium:0 mg

Cinnamon Apples

Prep time: 10 mins | Servings: 4

Ingredients:
- 1 tbsp. cinnamon powder
- 4 tbsps. raisins
- 4 cored big apples

Directions:
1. Stuff the apples while using the raisins, sprinkle the cinnamon, stick them inside a baking dish, introduce inside oven at 375 °F, bake for 20 minutes and serve cold.
2. Enjoy!

Nutritional Information:
Calories: 200, Fat:3 g, Carbs:8 g, Protein:5 g, Sugars:26 g, Sodium:120 mg

Green Tea Cream

Prep time: 1 hour |Servings: 6

Ingredients:
- 2 tbsps. green tea extract powder
- 3 tbsps. coconut sugar
- 14 oz. coconut milk
- 14 oz. coconut cream

Directions:
1. Put the milk in the very pan, add sugar and green tea herb powder, stir, give your simmer, cook for two minutes, remove heat, cool down, add coconut cream, whisk well, divide into small bowls whilst from the fridge for just two hours before serving.
2. Enjoy!

Nutritional Information:
Calories: 160, Fat:3 g, Carbs:7 g, Protein:6 g, Sugars:20 g, Sodium:45 mg

Coconut Figs

Prep time: 6 mins | Servings: 4

Ingredients:
- 12 halved figs
- 1 c. toasted and chopped almonds
- 2 tbsps. coconut butter
- ¼ c. coconut sugar

Directions:
1. Put butter inside the pot, get hot over medium heat, add sugar, whisk well, include almonds and figs, toss, cook for 5 minutes, divide into small cups and serve cold.
2. Enjoy!

Nutritional Information:
Calories: 150, Fat:4 g, Carbs:7 g, Protein:4 g, Sugars:12 g, Sodium:15 mg

Cocoa Banana Dessert Smoothie

Prep time: 5 mins | Servings: 2

Ingredients:
- ½ pitted, peeled and mashed big avocado
- 2 tsps. powered cocoa
- 2 peeled medium bananas
- ¾ c. almond milk

Directions:
1. In your blender, combine the bananas with the cocoa, avocado and milk, pulse well, divide into 2 glasses and serve.
2. Enjoy!

Nutritional Information:
Calories: 155, Fat:3 g, Carbs:6 g, Protein:5 g, Sugars:17 g, Sodium:66 mg

Chocolate Pomegranate Fudge

Prep time: 1 hour | Servings: 6

Ingredients:
- 1 tsp. vanilla flavoring
- 1 ½ c. chopped chocolate brown
- ½ c. coconut milk
- ½ c. pomegranate seeds
- ½ c. chopped almonds

Directions:
1. Put milk in a very pan, get hot over medium-low heat, add chocolate, stir well, cook for 5 minutes, remove heat, combine with all the vanilla flavoring, 50 % from the pomegranate seeds and 50 % of the almonds, stir well, spread on the lined baking sheet, sprinkle the rest using the almonds and pomegranate seeds, keep within the fridge for just two hours, cut and serve.
2. Enjoy!

Nutritional Information:
Calories: 148, Fat:3 g, Carbs:6 g, Protein:5 g, Sugars:3 g, Sodium:500 mg

Cashew Nut Cuppas

Prep time: 15 mins | Servings: 12

Ingredients:
- 15 g coconut cream
- 85 g maple syrup
- 30 g mini dark chocolate chips.
- 255 g unsalted cashew butter
- 5 g vanilla extract
- 70 g coconut oil

Directions:
1. Preheat oven to about 400 °F.
2. In a large bowl, add the cashew butter, coconut cream, coconut oil, vanilla and maple syrup, mix well.

3. Once the mixture is smooth, grease a cupcake pan, set with liners and set aside.
4. Carefully fold in the mini-chocolate chips, remember to always fold, or else you'll end up with runny chocolate which isn't' necessarily the worst thing in the world, but still, aesthetics right?
5. Pour into pan molds, and freeze.
6. Serve whenever the cups seem to have solidified, a couple hours in the deep is perfect!

Nutritional Information:
Calories: 163, Fat:11.9 g, Carbs:13 g, Protein:3 g, Sugars:1.7 g, Sodium:3.4 mg

Cheese Stuffed Apples

Prep Time: 20-25 min. | Servings: 4

Ingredients:
- 1 tbsp. raisins
- 1 whisked egg
- 8 oz. cottage cheese
- 1 tsp. confectioners' sugar
- 2 tbsps. honey
- 4 cored apples

Directions:
1. Preheat the oven to 400 °F.
2. In a mixing bowl, thoroughly mix the egg, cheese, honey, and raisins.
3. Spoon some flesh from the core part of the apples and fill with the cheese mix.
4. Bake for 18-20 minutes; top with confectioner's sugar and serve.

Nutritional Information:
Calories: 194, Fat:5.2 g, Carbs:23.8 g, Protein:3.6 g, Sugars:7 g, Sodium: 280mg

Green Apple Bowls

Prep time: 10 mins | Servings: 3

Ingredients:
- 1 tbsp. coconut sugar
- ½ tsp. vanilla flavoring
- 1 c. halved strawberries
- 3 cored and cubed big green apples
- ½ tsp. cinnamon powder

Directions:
1. In a bowl, combine the apples with strawberries, sugar, cinnamon and vanilla, toss and serve.
2. Enjoy!

Nutritional Information:
Calories: 205, Fat: 1 g, Carbs:8 g, Protein:4 g, Sugars:95 g, Sodium:9 mg

Peach Dip

Prep time: 10 mins | Servings: 2

Ingredients:
- 1 c. chopped peaches
- ½ c. nonfat yogurt
- ¼ tsp. ground nutmeg
- ¼ tsp. cinnamon powder

Directions:
1. In a bowl, combine the yogurt while using the peaches, cinnamon and nutmeg, whisk, divide into small bowls and serve being a snack.
2. Enjoy!

Nutritional Information:
Calories: 165, Fat:2 g, Carbs:14 g, Protein:13 g, Sugars:2 g, Sodium:2 mg

Pecan Granola

Prep time: 5 mins | Servings: 10

Ingredients:
- 50 g maple syrup
- ½ g nutmeg
- 2 ½ g salt
- 1400 g raw pecans
- 2 ½ g cayenne pepper
- 5 g ground cinnamon

Directions:
1. Preheat oven to about 400 °F.
2. In a large bowl, mix the pecans maple syrup, and spices, and toss till perfectly coated.
3. Spread out nuts on a baking sheet and roast for about 10 minutes.
4. Cool for another 10 minutes, then store or serve.

Nutritional Information:
Calories: 174, Fat:100.8 g, Carbs:23 g, Protein:13 g, Sugars:7 g, Sodium:135 mg

Walnut Green Beans

Prep time: 15-20 mins | Servings: 2-3

Ingredients:
- 2 c. roughly cut green beans
- 1 tbsp. olive oil
- 3 minced garlic cloves
- ½ c. chopped walnuts

Directions:
1. In a cooking pot, add and boil the beans in salted water until tender.
2. In a saucepan, add the beans, garlic, oil, and walnuts; cook for about 5-7 minutes stirring constantly.
3. Serve warm.

Nutritional Information:
Calories: 130, Fat:7 g, Carbs:15 g, Protein:5 g, Sugars:0 g, Sodium:104 mg

Banana Sashimi

Prep time: 5 mins| Servings: 1

Ingredients:
- ¼ tsp. chia seeds
- 15 g almond butter
- 1 medium banana

Directions:
1. Peel banana and cover one side in the nut butter, while placing it face up.
2. Slice banana evenly into even 1-centimeter thick pieces.
3. Sprinkle on toppings and serve!

Nutritional Information:
Calories: 194, Fat:8 g, Carbs:30 g, Protein:5 g, Sugars:0 g, Sodium:43 mg

Maple Malt

Prep time: 10 mins | Servings: 2

Ingredients:
- 2 ½ g vanilla essence
- 45 g maple syrup
- 5 g cinnamon
- 30 g chocolate
- 45 g cocoa powder
- 340 g almond milk

Directions:
1. Literally just pour it all into a saucepan and boil till it thickens.

Nutritional Information:
Calories: 1180, Fat:85.8 g, Carbs:80 g, Protein:40 g, Sugars:13 g, Sodium:0 mg

Parmesan Roasted Chickpeas

Prep time: 10 mins | Servings: 12

Ingredients:
- 1 tsp. thyme
- 2 crushed and minced garlic cloves
- 4 c. cooked garbanzo beans
- ½ c. fresh grated parmesan cheese
- 2 tbsps. olive oil

Directions:
1. Preheat oven to 400°F.
2. Pat dry the garbanzo beans to remove as much moisture as possible.
3. Place the garbanzo beans in bowl and combine with olive oil, garlic, thyme, and Parmesan cheese.
4. Spread the beans out on a baking sheet and place in the oven.
5. Bake for approximately 1 hour, tossing once halfway through.
6. Remove from oven and let cool before enjoying.

Nutritional Information:
Calories: 134.1, Fat:4.4 g, Carbs:18.3 g, Protein:5.7 g, Sugars:1 g, Sodium:202 mg

Apricot Nibbles

Prep time: 10 mins | Servings: 4

Ingredients:
- 1 tbsp. chopped pecans
- 2 tbsps. goat cheese
- Honey
- 12 dried apricots
- 1 tsp. rosemary
- 2 tbsps. blue cheese

Directions:
1. In a bowl, combine the pecans, goat cheese, blue cheese, and rosemary. Mix well. If you desire a creamier texture, place in the blender and pulse until smooth.
2. Add a dollop to the top of each dried apricot.
3. Serve with drizzled honey, if desired.

Nutritional Information:
Calories: 13.6, Fat:5.0 g, Carbs:20.8 g, Protein:4.1 g, Sugars:24 g, Sodium:5 mg

All Dressed Crispy Potato Skins

Prep time: 10 mins | Servings: 2

Ingredients:
- Butter-flavored cooking spray
- 1/8 tsp. freshly ground black pepper
- 1 tbsp. minced fresh rosemary
- 2 medium russet potatoes

Directions:
1. Preheat the oven to 375 °F.
2. Wash the potatoes with fresh water.
3. Pierce the potatoes with a fork.
4. Bake the potatoes in an oven about 1 hour or until the skins are crisp.
5. Cut the hot potatoes in half and scoop out most of the flesh, leaving about 1/8 inch from the skin.
6. Use a butter-flavored cooking spray to spray the insides of each potato skin.
7. Press rosemary and pepper into the potato skin.
8. Bake the potato skins again for another 5 to 10 minutes.
9. Serve immediately.

Nutritional Information:
Calories: 92.3, Fat:3.8 g, Carbs:9.6 g, Protein:4.6 g, Sugars:3.4 g, Sodium:803 mg

Delightful Coconut Shrimp

Prep time: 10 mins | Servings: 3

Ingredients:
- ¼ c. coconut milk
- 2 tbsps. panko breadcrumbs
- 2 tbsps. sweetened coconut
- 6 peeled and deveined large shrimp
- ¼ tsp. kosher salt

Directions:
1. Preheat your oven to 375 °F. Spray a baking sheet lightly with cooking spray.
2. Add the panko, coconut, and salt to a blender and run until the mixture has an even consistency.
3. Transfer the mixture to a small bowl. Then, pour the coconut milk into a separate small bowl.
4. Dip your shrimps in the coconut milk and then in the panko mixture one by one and place on the coated baking sheet.
5. Spray the top of the shrimps lightly with cooking spray. Bake the coated shrimps in the oven for about ten to fifteen minutes or until golden brown.

Nutritional Information:
Calories: 75, Fat:4 g, Carbs:4 g, Protein:5 g, Sugars:18 g, Sodium:450 mg

Creamy Peanuts with Apples

Prep time: 10 mins | Servings: 2

Ingredients:
- 4 oz. fat-free cream cheese
- 1 tbsp. diced peanuts
- ¼ c. orange juice
- 2 cored and sliced medium apples
- 1 tbsp. brown sugar
- ¾ tsp. vanilla

Directions:
1. Set your cream cheese on the counter for about five minutes to soften it.
2. Make the dip by mixing the cream cheese, vanilla, and brown sugar in a bowl. Add peanuts and mix until combined.
3. Add the sliced apples in a separate bowl and drizzle with orange juice to stop the apples from turning brown.
4. Serve the apples with the dip and enjoy!

Nutritional Information:
Calories: 110, Fat:2 g, Carbs:18 g, Protein:5 g, Sugars:3 g, Sodium:140 mg

Chapter 9 Stews and Soups

Vegetarian Split Pea Soup in a Crock Pot

Prep: 10 mins | Servings: 8

Ingredients:
- 2 chopped ribs celery
- 2 cubes low-sodium bouillon
- 8 c. water
- 2 c. uncooked green split peas
- 3 bay leaves
- 2 carrots
- 2 chopped potatoes
- Pepper and salt

Directions:
1. In your Crock-Pot, put the bouillon cubes, split peas, and water. Stir a bit to break up the bouillon cubes.
2. Next, add the chopped potatoes, celery, and carrots followed with bay leaves.
3. Stir to combine well.
4. Cover and cook for at least 4 hours on your Crock-Pot's low setting or until the green split peas are soft.
5. Add a bit salt and pepper as needed.
6. Before serving, remove the bay leaves and enjoy.

Nutritional Information:
Calories: 149, Fat:1 g, Carbs:30 g, Protein:7 g, Sugars:3 g, Sodium:732 mg

Rhubarb Stew

Prep time: 10 mins | Servings: 3

Ingredients:
- 1 tsp. grated lemon zest
- 1 ½ c. coconut sugar
- Juice of 1 lemon
- 1 ½ c. water
- 4 ½ c. roughly chopped rhubarbs

Directions:
1. In a pan, combine the rhubarb while using water, fresh lemon juice, lemon zest and coconut sugar, toss, bring using a simmer over medium heat, cook for 5 minutes, and divide into bowls and serve cold.
2. Enjoy!

Nutritional Information:
Calories: 108, Fat:1 g, Carbs:8 g, Protein:5 g, Sugars:2 g, Sodium:0 mg

Tofu Soup

Prep time: 10 mins | Servings: 8

Ingredients:
- 1 lb. cubed extra-firm tofu
- 3 diced medium carrots
- 8 c. low-sodium vegetable broth
- ½ tsp. freshly ground white pepper
- 8 minced garlic cloves
- 6 sliced and divided scallions
- 4 oz. sliced mushrooms
- 1-inch minced fresh ginger piece

Directions:
1. Pour the broth into a stockpot. Add all of the ingredients except for the tofu and last 2 scallions. Bring to a boil over high heat.
2. Once boiling, add the tofu. Reduce heat to low, cover, and simmer for 5 minutes.
3. Remove from heat, ladle soup into bowls, and garnish with the remaining sliced scallions. Serve immediately.

Nutritional Information:
Calories: 91, Fat:3 g, Carbs:8 g, Protein:6 g, Sugars:4 g, Sodium:900 mg

Easy Beef Stew

Prep time: 10 mins | Servings: 6

Ingredients:
- 1 shredded green cabbage head
- 4 chopped carrots
- 2 ½ lbs. non-fat beef brisket
- 3 chopped garlic cloves
- Black pepper
- 2 bay leaves
- 4 c. low-sodium beef stock

Directions:
1. Put the beef brisket in a pot, add stock, pepper, garlic and bay leaves, provide your simmer over medium heat and cook for an hour.
2. Add carrots and cabbage, stir, cook for a half-hour more, divide into bowls and serve for lunch.
3. Enjoy!

Nutritional Information:
Calories: 271, Fat:8 g, Carbs:16 g, Protein:9 g, Sugars:3.4 g, Sodium:760 mg

Zucchini-Basil Soup

Prep time: 10 mins | Servings: 5

Ingredients:
- 1/3 c. packed basil leaves
- ¾ c. chopped onion
- ¼ c. olive oil
- 2 lbs. trimmed and sliced zucchini
- 2 chopped garlic cloves
- 4 c. divided water

Directions:
1. Peel and julienne the skin from half of zucchini; toss with 1/2 teaspoon salt and drain in a sieve until wilted, at least 20 minutes. Coarsely chop remaining zucchini.
2. Cook onion and garlic in oil in a saucepan over medium-low heat, stirring occasionally, until onions are translucent. Add chopped zucchini and 1 teaspoon salt and cook, stirring occasionally.
3. Add 3 cups water and simmer with the lid ajar until tender. Pour the soup in a blender and purée soup with basil.
4. Bring remaining cup water to a boil in a small saucepan and blanch julienned zucchini. Drain.
5. Top soup with julienned zucchini. Season soup with salt and pepper and serve.

Nutritional Information:
Calories: 169.3, Fat:13.7 g, Carbs:12 g, Protein:2 g, Sugars:3.8 g, Sodium:8 mg

Black Bean Soup

Prep time: 10 mins | Servings: 4

Ingredients:
- 1 tsp. cinnamon powder
- 32 oz. low-sodium chicken stock
- 1 chopped yellow onion
- 1 chopped sweet potato
- 38 oz. no-salt-added, drained and rinsed canned black beans
- 2 tsps. organic olive oil

Directions:
1. Heat up a pot using the oil over medium heat, add onion and cinnamon, stir and cook for 6 minutes.
2. Add black beans, stock and sweet potato, stir, cook for 14 minutes, puree utilizing an immersion blender, divide into bowls and serve for lunch.
3. Enjoy!

Nutritional Information:
Calories: 221, Fat:3 g, Carbs:15 g, Protein:7 g, Sugars:4 g, Sodium:511 mg

Chicken and Dill Soup

Prep time: 10 mins | Servings: 6

Ingredients:
- 1 c. chopped yellow onion
- 1 whole chicken
- 1 lb. sliced carrots
- 6 c. low-sodium veggie stock
- ¼ tsp. black pepper and salt
- ½ c. chopped red onion
- 2 tsps. chopped dill

Directions:
1. Put chicken in a pot, add water to pay for, give your boil over medium heat, cook first hour, transfer to a cutting board, discard bones, shred the meat, strain the soup, get it back on the pot, heat it over medium heat and add the chicken.
2. Also add the carrots, yellow onion, red onion, a pinch of salt, black pepper and also the dill, cook for fifteen minutes, ladle into bowls and serve.
3. Enjoy!

Nutritional Information:
Calories: 202, Fat:6 g, Carbs:8 g, Protein:12 g, Sugars:6 g, Sodium:514 mg

Cherry Stew

Prep time: 10 mins | Servings: 6

Ingredients:
- 2 c. water
- ½ c. powered cocoa
- ¼ c. coconut sugar
- 1 lb. pitted cherries

Directions:
1. In a pan, combine the cherries with all the water, sugar plus the hot chocolate mix, stir, cook over medium heat for ten minutes, divide into bowls and serve cold.
2. Enjoy!

Nutritional Information:
Calories: 207, Fat:1 g, Carbs:8 g, Protein:6 g, Sugars:27 g, Sodium:19 mg

Sirloin Carrot Soup

Prep time: 30-35 mins | Servings: 4

Ingredients:
- 1 lb. chopped carrots and celery mix
- 32 oz. low-sodium beef stock
- 1/3 c. whole-wheat flour
- 1 lb. ground beef sirloin
- 1 tbsp. olive oil
- 1 chopped yellow onion

Directions:
1. Heat up the olive oil in a saucepan over medium-high flame; add the beef and the flour.
2. Stir well and cook to brown for 4-5 minutes.
3. Add the celery, onion, carrots, and stock; stir and bring to a simmer.
4. Turn down the heat to low and cook for 12-15 minutes.
5. Serve warm.

Nutritional Information:
Calories: 140, Fat:4.5 g, Carbs:16 g, Protein:9 g, Sugars:3 g, Sodium:670 mg

Easy Wonton Soup

Prep time: 5 mins | Servings: 8

Ingredients:
- 4 sliced scallions
- ¼ tsp. ground white pepper
- 2 c. sliced fresh mushrooms
- 4 minced garlic cloves
- 6 oz. dry whole-grain yolk-free egg noodles
- ½ lb. lean ground pork
- 1 tbsp. minced fresh ginger
- 8 c. low-sodium chicken broth

Directions:
1. Place a stockpot over medium heat. Add the ground pork, ginger, and garlic and sauté for 5 minutes. Drain any excess fat, then return to stovetop.
2. Add the broth and bring to a boil. Once boiling, stir in the mushrooms, noodles, and white pepper. Cover and simmer for 10 minutes.
3. Remove pot from heat. Stir in the scallions and serve immediately.

Nutritional Information:
Calories: 143, Fat:4 g, Carbs:14 g, Protein:12 g, Sugars:0.8 g, Sodium:901 mg

Sweet Potato Soup

Prep time: 10 mins | Servings: 6

Ingredients:
- 28 oz. veggie stock
- 4 big sweet potatoes
- ¼ tsp. black pepper
- 1/3 c. low-sodium heavy cream
- ¼ tsp. ground nutmeg

Directions:
1. Arrange the sweet potatoes around the lined baking sheet, bake them at 350 °F for 60 minutes and thirty minutes, cool them down, peel, roughly chop them and put them inside the pot.
2. Add stock, nutmeg, cream and pepper, pulse effectively utilizing an immersion blender, heat the soup over medium heat, cook for 10 minutes, ladle into bowls and serve.
3. Enjoy!

Nutritional Information:
Calories: 235, Fat:4 g, Carbs:16 g, Protein:18 g, Sugars:10 g, Sodium:800 mg

Omnipotent Organic Chicken Thigh Soup

Prep time: 5 mins | Servings: 4

Ingredients:
- 1 c. fresh pineapple chunks
- 1 tsp. cinnamon
- ½ c. chopped up green onion
- 2 tbsps. coconut aminos
- 2 lbs. organic chicken thigh
- 1/8 tsp. flavored vinegar
- ½ c. coconut cream

Directions:
1. Set your pot to Sauté mode and add ghee
2. Allow the ghee to melt and add diced up onion, cook for about 5 minutes until the onions are caramelized
3. Add pressed garlic, ham, broth and simmer for 2-3 minutes
4. Add thyme and asparagus and lock up the lid
5. Cook on SOUP mode for 45 minutes
6. Release the pressure naturally and enjoy!

Nutritional Information:
Calories: 161, Fat:8 g, Carbs:16 g, Protein:6 g, Sugars:0.7 g, Sodium:307 mg

Minty Grapefruit Stew

Prep time: 10 mins | Servings: 6

Ingredients:
- 1 c. coconut sugar
- 4 peeled and roughly chopped grapefruits
- ½ c. chopped mint
- 1 c. water

Directions:
1. Put water in a very pan, add sugar, mint and grapefruits, toss, bring to a simmer over medium heat, cook for ten minutes, divide into bowls and serve cold.
2. Enjoy!

Nutritional Information:
Calories: 120, Fat:1 g, Carbs:2 g, Protein:6 g, Sugars:20 g, Sodium:4 mg

Apple Butternut Soup

Prep time: 10 mins | Servings: 6

Ingredients:
- 2 c. diced apple
- 1/8 tsp. ground allspice
- 6 c. diced butternut squash
- 6 c. water
- ½ tsp. ground cinnamon
- 2 c. unsweetened apple juice

Directions:
1. Place diced squash and apple into a stockpot, add the water and apple juice, and bring to a boil over high heat. Once boiling, reduce heat to medium-low, cover, and simmer until tender, roughly 20 minutes.
2. Remove from heat. Add spices and stir to combine. Purée in a blender or food processor.
3. Serve warm.

Nutritional Information:
Calories: 150, Fat:0 g, Carbs:38 g, Protein:3 g, Sugars:6.5 g, Sodium:409 mg

Beef Soup

Prep time: 10 mins | Servings: 4

Ingredients:
- 1 lb. chopped mixed carrots and celery
- 32 oz. low-sodium beef stock
- 1 lb. ground beef sirloin
- 1 tbsp. extra virgin olive oil
- 1 chopped yellow onion
- 1/3 c. whole-wheat grains flour

Directions:
1. Heat up a pot while using the oil over medium-high heat, add beef and flour, stir well and brown for 5 minutes.
2. Add onion, carrots, celery and stock, stir, provide a simmer, reduce heat to medium, cook the soup for quarter-hour, ladle into bowls and serve for lunch.
3. Enjoy!

Nutritional Information:
Calories: 281, Fat:3 g, Carbs:14 g, Protein:11 g, Sugars:1.4 g, Sodium:167 mg

Strawberry Soup a La Kiev

Prep time: 31 mins | Servings: 8

Ingredients:
- 1 c. brown sugar
- 1 c. favorite red wine
- 3 c. chopped strawberries
- 1 c. sour cream
- 4 c cold water

Directions:
1. In a food processor, blend the strawberries.
2. Pour the mixture in a medium sauce pan.
3. Stir in the brown sugar, sour cream, wine and water.

4. Cook over low heat. Stir gently for 20 minutes. Do not allow the soup to boil, just serve it warm.

Nutritional Information:
Calories: 37, Fat:0.9 g, Carbs:19 g, Protein:8 g, Sugars:11 g, Sodium:25 mg

Summer Strawberry Stew

Prep time: 10 mins | Servings: 6

Ingredients:
- 2 tbsps. water
- ¼ tsp. almond extract
- 2 tbsps. fresh lemon juice
- 16 oz. halved strawberries
- 2 tbsps. coconut sugar
- 2 tbsps. cornstarch

Directions:
1. In a pot, combine the strawberries because of the water, sugar, fresh lemon juice, cornstarch and almond extract, toss well, cook over medium heat for ten minutes, divide into bowls and serve.
2. Enjoy!

Nutritional Information:
Calories: 160, Fat:2 g, Carbs:6 g, Protein:6 g, Sugars:27 g, Sodium:55 mg

Peach Stew

Prep time: 10 mins | Servings: 6

Ingredients:
- 3 tbsps. coconut sugar
- 5 c. peeled and cubed peaches
- 2 c. water
- 1 tsp. grated ginger

Directions:
1. In a pot, combine the peaches while using the sugar, ginger and water, toss, provide a boil over medium heat, cook for ten minutes, divide into bowls and serve cold.
2. Enjoy!

Nutritional Information:
Calories: 142, Fat:1 g, Carbs:7 g, Protein:2 g, Sugars:2 g, Sodium:1 mg

Eggplant Soup

Prep time: 10 mins | Servings: 4

Ingredients:
- 2 tbsps. no-salt-added tomato paste
- 1 tbsp. olive oil
- 1 quart low-sodium veggie stock
- ¼ tsp. black pepper
- 1 chopped red onion
- 2 roughly cubed big eggplants
- 1 tbsp. chopped cilantro

Directions:
1. Heat up a pot with the oil over medium heat, add the onion, stir and sauté for 5 minutes.
2. Add the eggplants and the other ingredients, bring to a simmer over medium heat, cook for 25 minutes, divide into bowls and serve.

Nutritional Information:
Calories: 335, Fat:14.4 g, Carbs:16.1 g, Protein:8.4 g, Sugars:5 g, Sodium: 375 mg

Blueberry Stew

Prep time: 10 mins | Servings: 4

Ingredients:
- 1 c. water
- 2 tbsps. lemon juice
- 12 oz. blueberries
- 3 tbsps. coconut sugar

Directions:
1. In a pan, combine the blueberries with the sugar and the other ingredients, bring to a gentle simmer and cook over medium heat for 10 minutes.
2. Divide into bowls and serve.

Nutritional Information:
Calories: 122, Fat:0.4 g, Carbs:26.7 g, Protein:1.5 g, Sugars:15 g, Sodium:10 mg

Leek and Chicken Soup

Prep time: 15 mins | Servings: 4

Ingredients:
- ½ c. freshly squeezed lemon juice
- 3 roughly chopped leek
- 1 sliced whole chicken
- 12 c. low-sodium veggie stock
- 3 tbsps. organic olive oil
- ¼ tsp. salt and black pepper
- 2 c. chopped yellow onion

Directions:
1. Put chicken in a very pot, add the stock, a pinch of salt and black pepper, stir, provide a boil over medium heat and skim foam.
2. Add leeks, toss and simmer for an hour or so.
3. Heat up a pan with the oil over medium heat, add onion, stir and cook for 5 minutes.
4. Add this towards pot, also add the freshly squeezed lemon juice, toss, cook for twenty minutes more, ladle into bowls and serve.
5. Enjoy!

Nutritional Information:
Calories: 199, Fat:3 g, Carbs:6 g, Protein:11 g, Sugars:6 g, Sodium:446 mg

Courgette, Pea & Pesto Soup

Prep time: 10 mins | Servings: 4

Ingredients:
- 1 sliced garlic clove
- 400g drained and rinsed cannellini beans
- 1 tbsp. olive oil
- 200g frozen peas
- 2 tbsps. basil pesto
- 500g quartered courgettes
- 1lb. hot vegetable stock

Directions:
1. Heat the oil in a large saucepan. Cook the garlic for a few seconds, then add the courgettes and cook for 3 minutes until they start to soften. Stir in the peas and cannellini beans, pour on the hot stock and cook for a further 3 minutes.
2. Stir the pesto through the soup with some seasoning, then ladle into bowls and serve with crusty brown bread, if you like. Or pop in a flask to take to work.

Nutritional Information:
Calories: 200, Fat:8 g, Carbs:21 g, Protein:12 g, Sugars:7 g, Sodium:414 mg

Watermelon Stew

Prep time: 5 mins | Servings: 4

Ingredients:
- 1 tsp. grated lime zest
- 1 ½ c. water
- Juice of 1 lime
- 1 ½ c. coconut sugar
- 4 c. peeled and sliced watermelon

Directions:
1. In a pan, combine the watermelon with the lime zest, and the other ingredients, toss, bring to a simmer over medium heat, cook for 8 minutes, divide into bowls and serve cold.

Nutritional Information:
Calories: 233, Fat:0.2 g, Carbs:61.5 g, Protein:0.9 g, Sugars:10 g, Sodium:53 mg

Apricots Stew

Prep time: 10 mins | Servings: 4

Ingredients:
- 2 tbsps. lemon juice
- 2 c. halved apricots
- 2 tbsps. coconut sugar
- 2 c. water

Directions:

1. In a pot, combine the apricots with the water and the other ingredients, toss, cook over medium heat for 15 minutes, divide into bowls and serve.

Nutritional Information:
Calories: 260, Fat:6.2 g, Carbs:5.6 g, Protein:6 g, Sugars:9 g, Sodium:2 mg

Grapes Stew

Prep time: 10 mins | Servings: 4

Ingredients:
- 2 tbsps. coconut sugar
- 2 tsps. cardamom powder
- 1 c. green grapes
- 1 ½ c. water
- Juice of ½ lime

Directions:
1. Heat up a pan with the water medium heat, add the grapes and the other ingredients, bring to a simmer, cook for 20 minutes, divide into bowls and serve.

Nutritional Information:
Calories: 384, Fat: 12.5 g, Carbs:13.8 g, Protein:5.6 g, Sugars:15.4 g, Sodium:2 mg

Zucchini Cream Soup

Prep time: 10 mins | Servings: 4

Ingredients:
- 1 tbsp. chopped dill
- 1 tbsp. olive oil
- 32 oz. low-sodium chicken stock
- 1 tsp. grated ginger
- 1 lb. chopped zucchinis
- 1 c. coconut cream
- 1 chopped yellow onion

Directions:
1. Heat up a pot with the oil over medium heat, add the onion and ginger, stir and cook for 5 minutes.
2. Add the zucchinis and the other ingredients, bring to a simmer and cook over medium heat for 15 minutes.
3. Blend using an immersion blender, divide into bowls and serve.

Nutritional Information:
Calories: 293, Fat:12.3 g, Carbs:11.2 g, Protein:6.4 g, Sugars:5.2 g, Sodium:443 mg

Beef Prune Stew

Prep time: 65-70 mins | Servings: 4-5

Ingredients:
- 1 diced onion
- ½ c. water
- 1 c. prunes
- 1 diced parsley
- 1 lb. beef stew meat
- ½ c. tomato sauce

Directions:
1. In a cooking pot, boil the beef in the unsalted water until half-cooked. Set aside.
2. In a saucepan; add the oil, onions, and parsley.
3. Cook over medium-high flame to soften.
4. Add the beef, tomato sauce, and water to the saucepan; stir well.
5. Add the prunes, cover and simmer the mix until the beef is tender, for approximately 30-40 minutes.
6. Serve warm.

Nutritional Information:
Calories: 338, Fat:4.4 g, Carbs:11.9 g, Protein:10.7 g, Sugars:25 g, Sodium:47 mg

Chapter 10 Salads and Sauces

New Potato Salad

Prep time: 20 mins | Servings: 4

Ingredients:
- ¼ c. chopped green onions
- 1 tsp. dried dill
- Black pepper
- 16 washed, boiled and quartered small potatoes
- 2 tbsps. olive oil

Directions:
1. In a salad bowl combine all the ingredients and mix well.

Nutritional Information:
Calories: 196, Fat:6 g, Carbs:28 g, Protein:6.7 g, Sugars:1.9 g, Sodium:71 mg

Potato & Octopus Salad

Prep time: 10 mins | Servings: 6-8

Ingredients:
- 2 lbs. octopus
- 2 crushed garlic cloves
- 1 bay leaf
- ½ tbsp. peppercorns
- 2 lbs. potatoes
- 1 chopped parsley bunch
- 1 whole garlic cloves
- ½ c. olive oil
- 5 tbsps. White wine vinegar

Directions:
1. Scrub the potatoes well and place them unpeeled and whole in your pressure cooker. Pour in enough water to cover the potatoes halfway. Close and lock the lid of your pressure cooker. Cook on low pressure for 15 minutes.
2. Once the cooking time is up, release the pressure using the quick release method and take the potatoes out of the pressure cooker. Don't discard the cooking liquid.
3. Peel the hot potatoes; dice them into small cubes and place in a large mixing bowl.
4. To cook the prepared octopus in the pressure cooker, pour enough water to almost cover it.
5. Add the bay leaf, whole garlic clove, and peppercorns and bring to the boil. Then add the octopus.
6. Close and lock the lid. Cook on low pressure for 15 minutes. When the time is up, release the pressure using the quick release method.
7. Once the octopus is done, take it out of the pressure cooker and remove any remaining skin.
8. Add the octopus chunks to the bowl with the potatoes and mix well.
9. To prepare the vinaigrette, combine all the ingredients in a jar and shake well to blend everything.
10. Flood the octopus and potato chunks with the vinaigrette, garnish with the chopped parsley and serve.

Nutritional Information:
Calories: 119, Fat:0 g, Carbs:27 g, Protein:3 g, Sugars:1.8 g, Sodium:266 mg

Balsamic Beet Salad

Prep time: 5 mins | Servings: 4

Ingredients:
- Extra virgin olive oil
- Kosher flavored vinegar
- 6 medium sized beets
- Freshly ground black pepper
- 1 c. water
- Balsamic vinegar

Directions:
1. Wash the beets carefully and trim them to ½ inch portions
2. Add 1 cup of water to the pot
3. Place a steamer on top and arrange the beets on top of the steamer
4. Lock up the lid and cook on HIGH pressure for 1 minute
5. Release the pressure naturally and allow the beet to cool
6. Slice the top of the skin carefully
7. Slice up the beets in uniform portions and season with flavored vinegar and pepper
8. Add a splash of balsamic vinegar and allow them to marinate for 30 minutes
9. Add a bit of extra olive oil and serve!

Nutritional Information:
Calories: 120, Fat:7 g, Carbs:13 g, Protein:2 g, Sugars:9 g, Sodium:330 mg

Mango Tango Salad

Prep time: 10 mins | Servings: 6

Ingredients:
- 1 juiced lime
- ½ seeded and minced jalapeno pepper
- 2 tbsps. chopped fresh cilantro leaves
- 3 pitted and cubed ripe mangoes
- 1 tsp. minced red onion

Directions:
1. Combine everything in a mixing bowl and let it rest ten minutes. Toss before serving.

Nutritional Information:
Calories: 68, Fat:0 g, Carbs:16 g, Protein:1 g, Sugars:15 g, Sodium:0 mg

Terrific Tortellini Salad

Prep time: 10 mins | Servings: 8

Ingredients:
- ½ c. bottled reduced-fat ranch salad dressing
- 3 c. broccoli florets
- 1 c. halved fresh pea pods
- 1 chopped large tomato
- 9 oz. refrigerated light cheese tortellini
- 1 c. medium sliced carrots
- ¼ c. sliced green onions

Directions:
1. In a large saucepan cook pasta according to package directions. Add the broccoli and carrots during the last 3 minutes of cooking. Drain.
2. Rinse with cold water and drain again.
3. In a large bowl combine the cooked pasta mixture and green onions; drizzle with dressing. Gently toss to coat. Cover and chill for 2 to 24 hours.
4. Before serving, gently stir tomato and pea pods into pasta mixture. If necessary, stir in a little milk to moisten.

Nutritional Information:
Calories: 378, Fat:28 g, Carbs:19 g, Protein:13 g, Sugars:1 g, Sodium:310 mg

Squash Garden Salad

Prep time: 15 mins | Servings: 2

Ingredients:
- 1 pitted and cubed avocado
- 2 tbsps. lemon juice
- 2 tbsps. olive oil
- 8 oz. peeled and cubed summer squash
- 1 oz. chopped watercress

Directions:
1. Arrange all the vegetables in a salad bowl and dress with olive oil and lemon juice.
2. Add the watercress leaves.

Nutritional Information:
Calories: 326, Fat:29.6 g, Carbs:3 g, Protein:3 g, Sugars:4 g, Sodium:320 mg

Beet, Prune and Walnut Salad

Prep time: 5 mins | Servings: 2

Ingredients:
- 1 minced garlic clove
- 2 tbsps. olive oil
- 10 chopped prunes
- 2 peeled and grated small beets
- 1 c. chopped walnuts

Directions:
1. Combine all the ingredients in a salad bowl.
2. Dress with olive oil.

Nutritional Information:
Calories: 296, Fat:21 g, Carbs:26 g, Protein:3.6 g, Sugars:17 g, Sodium:159 mg

Steamed Saucy Garlic Greens

Prep time: 5 mins | Servings: 4

Ingredients:
- 1/8 tsp. flavored vinegar
- 1 peeled whole clove
- ¼ c. water
- 1 tbsp. lemon juice
- 1 bunch leafy greens
- ½ c. soaked cashews
- 1 tsp. coconut aminos

Directions:
1. Make the sauce by draining and discard the soaking water from your cashew and add them cashew to blender
2. Add fresh water, lemon juice, flavored vinegar, coconut aminos, and garlic
3. Blitz until you have a smooth cream and transfer to bowl
4. Add ½ cup of water to the pot
5. Place the steamer basket to the pot and add the greens in the basket
6. Lock up the lid and steam for 1 minute
7. Quick release the pressure
8. Transfer the steamed greens to strainer and extract excess water
9. Place the greens into a mixing bowl
10. Add lemon garlic sauce and toss
11. Enjoy!

Nutritional Information:
Calories: 77, Fat:5 g, Carbs:0 g, Protein:2 g, Sugars:2 g, Sodium:534 mg

Scoop-It-Up Chicken Salad

Prep time: 10 mins | Servings: 1

Ingredients:
- 1 tbsp. salsa
- 2 tbsps. chopped celery
- 1/3 c. chopped cooked chicken
- 1 tbsp. light mayonnaise dressing
- 4 Mini taco shells
- 1 tbsp. shredded cheddar cheese

Directions:
1. In a small bowl combine chicken, celery, mayonnaise dressing, salsa, and cheese; toss to mix. Spoon into a container; cover tightly.
2. Wrap taco shells in plastic wrap. Pack chicken salad and taco shells in an insulated bag with an ice pack.
3. To serve, use taco shells to scoop up salad.

Nutritional Information:
Calories: 254, Fat:18 g, Carbs:3.3 g, Protein:19 g, Sugars6 g, Sodium:348 mg

Daikon Radish Salad

Prep time: 5 mins | Servings: 2

Ingredients:
- 2 tbsps. lemon juice
- 2 peeled and grated small daikons
- 3 tbsps. olive oil
- ¼ peeled and grated medium pumpkin
- 2 c. minced parsley

Directions:
1. Combine all the ingredients in a salad bowl.
2. Sprinkle with olive oil and lemon juice.

Nutritional Information:
Calories: 237, Fat:2.6 g, Carbs:13.9 g, Protein:2.0 g, Sugars:12 g, Sodium:350 mg

Boiled Carrot Salad with Green Peas

Prep time: 5 mins | Servings: 2

Ingredients:
- 1 tbsp. olive oil
- 2 whole carrots
- ½ c. canned green peas

Directions:
1. Boil the carrots in salted water for 20 min.
2. Cool, peel and cut into cubes.
3. Mix carrots with green peas in a salad bowl and dress with olive oil.

Nutritional Information:
Calories: 105, Fat:7.2 g, Carbs:28.1 g, Protein:8.6 g, Sugars:110 g, Sodium:5 mg

Faux Soy Sauce

Prep time: 2 mins | Servings: 3-4

Ingredients:
- 3 tbsps. unflavored rice wine vinegar
- 1 tsp. sodium-free beef bouillon granules
- ½ tsp. freshly ground black pepper
- ¼ c. molasses
- 1 tbsp. water

Directions:
1. Measure all the ingredients into a small saucepan or microwave-safe bowl and heat on low to combine, roughly 1 minute.
2. Use immediately or store in an airtight container and refrigerate until ready to use.

Nutritional Information:
Calories: 25, Fat:0 g, Carbs:6 g, Protein:0 g, Sugars:0.2 g, Sodium:900 mg

Citrus Shrimp Salad

Prep time: 10 mins | Servings: 4

Ingredients:
- ¼ c. freshly squeezed orange juice
- 6 c. spinach and lettuce mix
- 2 peeled and chopped oranges
- ½ lb. peeled and rinsed cooked small salad shrimp
- 1 tbsp. balsamic vinegar
- 1 chopped cucumber

Directions:
1. Combine the shrimp with the orange juice, vinegar and cucumber and toss.
2. Chill the mixture in the refrigerator for at least 30 minutes.
3. Place the mixture on top of the lettuce and spinach and sprinkle with orange segments.

Nutritional Information:
Calories: 125, Fat:0.8 g, Carbs:15.6 g, Protein:14.4 g, Sugars:8 g, Sodium:800 mg

Calamari Salad

Prep time: 15 mins | Servings: 2

Ingredients:
- 1 peeled and sliced cucumber
- Lettuce leaves
- 3 ½ oz. washed, cleaned and sliced calamari fillets
- Fresh parsley
- 1 peeled, boiled and sliced potato
- 1 tbsp. sour cream
- 1 peeled, cored and sliced apple

Directions:
1. Place the calamari into boiling salted water and cook for 5 min.
2. Arrange lettuce leaves on the bottom of a salad bowl. Mix the apple and vegetable strips with the calamari. Dress with sour cream, place on the lettuce leaves, and garnish with the parsley.

Nutritional Information:
Calories: 468, Fat:8.5 g, Carbs:5.1 g, Protein:17.8 g, Sugars:0.3 g, Sodium:50.9 mg

Shrimp and Asparagus Salad

Prep time: 10 mins | Servings: 4

Ingredients:
- 2 c. halved cherry tomatoes
- Cracked black pepper
- 12 oz. trimmed fresh asparagus spears
- 16 oz. frozen peeled and cooked shrimp
- Cracker bread
- 4 c. watercress
- ½ c. bottled light raspberry

Directions:
1. In a large skillet, cook asparagus, covered, in a small amount of boiling lightly salted water for 3 minutes or until crisp-tender; drain in a colander. Run under cold water until cool.
2. Divide asparagus among 4 dinner plates; top with watercress, shrimp, and cherry tomatoes. Drizzle with dressing.
3. Sprinkle with cracked black pepper and serve with cracker bread.

Nutritional Information:
Calories: 155.5, Fat:1.4 g, Carbs:15 g, Protein:22 g, Sugars:1 g, Sodium:324 mg

Carrot and Walnut Salad

Prep time: 10 mins | Servings: 2

Ingredients:
- ¼ c. chopped walnuts
- 1 peeled, cored and sliced apple
- Parsley leaves
- 1 peeled and grated carrot
- 1 tbsp. honey

Directions:
1. Coat the grated carrots with honey.
2. Arrange the carrots, apples and walnuts in a salad bowl.
3. Decorate with parsley leaves.

Nutritional Information:
Calories: 193, Fat:8.7 g, Carbs:27.2 g, Protein:1.4 g, Sugars:238 g, Sodium:632 mg

Pickled Onion Salad

Prep time: 1 hour | Servings: 4

Ingredients:
- 4 chopped spring onions
- ½ c. chopped fresh cilantro
- 2 tbsps. brown sugar
- 1 tbsp. lime juice
- ½ c. cider vinegar
- 2 thinly sliced red onions

- 4 lettuce leaves
- 2 tsps. olive oil

Directions:
1. In a salad bowl combine the onions, vinegar, oil and sugar.
2. Cover and refrigerate for 1 hr.
3. Add cilantro and lime juice.
4. Serve on lettuce leaves.

Nutritional Information:
Calories: 223, Fat:14.1 g, Carbs:20 g, Protein:1.8 g, Sugars:0 g, Sodium:0.5 mg

Chicken Raisin Salad

Prep time: 15-20 mins | Servings: 2

Ingredients:
- 2 tbsps. lemon juice
- 2 tbsps. raisins
- 1 peeled, cored and cubed apple
- ¼ c. chopped celery
- 2 tbsps. olive oil
- 3 ¼ c. skinless and sliced chicken meat

Directions:
1. In a saucepan or skillet, cook the cubed chicken meat in olive oil until golden.
2. Transfer the cooked meat to a mixing bowl of medium-large size and add all other ingredients. Stir to combine
3. Serve while the chicken is warm.

Nutritional Information:
Calories: 382, Fat:16 g, Carbs:41 g, Protein:25.7 g, Sugars:21 g, Sodium:125 mg

Pickled Grape Salad with Pear, Taleggio and Walnuts

Prep time: 15 mins| Servings: 3

Ingredients:
- 200g sliced taleggio cheese
- 4 tbsps. red wine vinegar
- 2 tbsps. light brown sugar
- 2 handfuls fresh watercress
- 100g halved red grapes
- 1 wedged pear
- 50g halved walnut

Directions:
1. Heat a cast-iron skillet or frying pan and toast the walnut halves, until they are slightly brown and give off a lovely nutty aroma. Set aside to cool.
2. Stir together the red wine vinegar and light brown sugar in a bowl, and leave for 5 minutes to allow the sugar to dissolve.
3. Add the grapes to this sweet and tangy mixture, and toss. Marinate for 10 minutes while you work on the rest of the recipe.
4. Scatter the watercress onto 3 plates or onto one large sharing platter, and then top evenly with the taleggio cheese and pear wedges.
5. Drain the grapes from their marinade, but do not discard the marinade.
6. Whisk 2 tablespoons of olive oil into the pickling marinade.
7. Scatter the pickled grapes all over the salad, and then drizzle over 3-4 tablespoons of the dressing.
8. Finish with the toasted walnut halves, and enjoy immediately.

Nutritional Information:
Calories: 421, Fat:28.4 g, Carbs:24.1 g, Protein:15.9 g, Sugars:23.9 g, Sodium:1 mg

Mango Salad

Prep time: 5 mins | Servings: 2

Ingredients:
- ½ seeded and minced jalapeño pepper
- 2 tbsps. chopped fresh cilantro
- Juice of 1 lime
- 3 pitted and cubed ripe mangos
- 1 tsp. minced red onion

Directions:

1. Combine all ingredients in a salad bowl.
2. Toss well.

Nutritional Information:
Calories: 331, Fat:5 g, Carbs:28.1 g, Protein:1 g, Sugars:27 g, Sodium:3.4 mg

Fresh Fruit Salad

Prep time: 15 mins | Servings: 3

Ingredients:
- 1 halved and sliced ripe banana
- 170 g sliced and halved strawberries,
- 170 g julienned granny smith apples
- 1 g salt
- 340 g chopped ripe pineapple
- 170 g sliced and quartered kiwi
- 340 g chopped ripe mango

Directions:
1. Cut the mangoes and kiwis into small cubes to get that full burst of flavor.
2. Slice the bananas about a centimeter thick and then halve them.
3. Once you have all the fruits cut up, put them in a bowl, and top with salt.
4. Stir it all together and you are ready to serve!

Nutritional Information:
Calories: 203, Fat:0.9 g, Carbs:51 g, Protein:2 g, Sugars:16 g, Sodium:26 mg

Dried Apricot Sauce

Prep time: 2 hours | Servings: 4

Ingredients:
- ½ c. sugar
- 4 oz. dried apricots
- 3½ tbsps. cornstarch

Directions:
1. Place the dried apricots into enough hot water to cover them and let soak for 1-2 hours.
2. Bring the water with dried apricots to a boil and cook on low heat for 30 minutes.
3. Add sugar and bring back to a boil, constantly stirring.
4. Prepare the cornstarch solution: add the cornstarch to water in a 1:4 ratio, mix well.
5. Add the cornstarch solution to the boiling dried apricot sauce. Stir and remove from heat after 5 minutes.
6. Serve as topping for your favorite desserts.

Nutritional Information:
Calories: 153, Fat:0.2 g, Carbs:3.8 g, Protein:0.5 g, Sugars:7 g, Sodium:0.7 mg

Tomato, Cucumber, and Basil Salad

Prep time: 10 mins | Serves 4

Ingredients:
- 1 minced garlic clove
- ¼ tsp. freshly ground black pepper
- 1 tbsp. olive oil
- 1 thinly sliced small onion
- 2 medium cucumbers
- 4 quartered ripe medium tomatoes
- ¼ c. chopped fresh basil
- 3 tbsps. red wine vinegar

Directions:
1. Peel the cucumbers, slice in half lengthwise, and then use a spoon to gently scrape out the seeds.
2. Slice the cucumber halves and place in a bowl. Add the tomatoes, onion, and basil.
3. Place the remaining ingredients into a small bowl and whisk well to combine.
4. Pour the dressing over the salad and toss to coat. Serve immediately or cover and refrigerate until ready to serve.

Nutritional Information:
Calories: 66, Fat:4 g, Carbs:7 g, Protein:1 g, Sugars:8 g, Sodium:15 mg

Strawberries and Avocado Salad

Prep time: 5 mins | Servings: 2

Ingredients:
- 2 c. halved strawberries
- 2 pitted and peeled avocados
- 3 tbsps. chopped mint
- 1 peeled and sliced banana

Directions:
1. In a bowl, combine the banana while using the strawberries, mint and avocados, toss and serve cold.
2. Enjoy!

Nutritional Information:
Calories:150 , Fat:4 g, Carbs:8 g, Protein:6 g, Sugars:2 g, Sodium:700 mg

Kelp Salad

Prep time: 15 mins | Servings: 2

Ingredients:
- ½ c. chopped spring onions
- ¼ shredded white cabbage head
- 1 oz. boiled kelp
- 1 tbsp. olive oil
- 1 peeled and sliced cucumber
- 1 hard-boiled and wedged egg

Directions:
1. Prepare the ingredients and combine them in a salad bowl.
2. Dress with olive oil.

Nutritional Information:
Calories: 162, Fat:9.8 g, Carbs:23 g, Protein:3 g, Sugars:1 g, Sodium:761 mg

Chicken Celery Salad

Prep time: 10 mins | Servings: 2

Ingredients:
- ¼ c. chopped celery
- 2 tbsps. olive oil
- 3¼ c. skinless cubed chicken meat
- 2 tbsps. raisins
- 1 peeled, cored and cubed apple
- 2 tbsps. lemon juice

Directions:
1. Preheat a non-stick pan and cook the chicken cubes in olive oil until golden.
2. In a salad bowl combine all the ingredients and dress with olive oil and lemon juice.

Nutritional Information:
Calories: 345, Fat:16.5 g, Carbs:16.7 g, Protein:10.7 g, Sugars:0.5 g, Sodium:191 mg

Garlic Potato Salad

Prep time: 10 mins | Servings: 6

Ingredients:
- ¼ c. olive oil
- 3 minced garlic cloves
- 2 tsps. chopped fresh rosemary
- Freshly ground black pepper
- 6 medium potatoes
- 1 c. sliced scallions
- 2 tbsps. unflavored rice vinegar

Directions:
1. Put the potatoes into a pot and add enough water to cover by 1 inch. Place over high heat and bring to a boil. Boil until fork tender but still solid; depending upon size, roughly 20 minutes.
2. Once cooked, remove from heat and place under cold running water. Drain and set potatoes aside to cool. Once cool enough to handle, cut into bite-sized cubes.

3. Place cubed potatoes, garlic, and scallions into a mixing bowl and toss to combine.
4. Measure the olive oil, vinegar, and rosemary into a small mixing bowl. Add freshly ground black pepper and whisk well to combine.
5. Pour the dressing over the salad and stir gently to coat. Serve immediately, or cover and refrigerate until serving.

Nutritional Information:
Calories: 204, Fat:9 g, Carbs:28 g, Protein:2 g, Sugars:6 g, Sodium:195 mg

Spring Salad

Prep time: 8 hours | Servings: 2

Ingredients:
- 1 bunch minced dill
- 7 oz. halved small radishes
- 3 halved cucumbers
- ½ c. water
- 3 tbsps. lemon juice
- ¼ c. presoaked skinless almonds
- 1 minced garlic clove
- 1 tsp. honey

Directions:
1. Soak the almonds in water overnight.
2. Using a blender mix the almonds with garlic, honey, lemon juice and water.
3. Arrange the cucumbers, radish and dill in a salad bowl and pour the almond-garlic dressing over the salad.

Nutritional Information:
Calories: 197, Fat:6.8 g, Carbs:4.4 g, Protein:2 g, Sugars:2 g, Sodium:15 mg

Appetizing Cucumber Salad

Prep time: 10 mins | Servings: 8

Ingredients:
- 1 peeled and minced garlic clove
- 1 tbsp. fresh lemon juice
- 2 peeled cucumber
- 2 tbsps. low-fat, low-sodium mayonnaise
- 1 tsp. mustard
- 1/3 c. roughly chopped fresh dill leaves
- ½ tsp. pepper
- ½ c. sour cream

Directions:
1. Slice cucumber into 3 equal lengths. Then slice lengthwise into quarters or smaller to create cucumber sticks. Drain in a colander and set aside.
2. In a medium bowl whisk well the remaining ingredients.
3. Add the drained cucumber into bowl of dressing and toss well to coat.
4. Serve and enjoy.

Nutritional Information:
Calories: 37.9, Fat:2.3 g, Carbs:3.3 g, Protein:1 g, Sugars:5 g, Sodium:246 mg

Pumpkin Salad

Prep time: 15 mins | Servings: 2

Ingredients:
- Juice of ½ lemon
- 2 tbsps. pumpkin seeds
- 2 oz. peeled, cored and sliced apples
- 1 tbsp. honey
- 2 oz. peeled and sliced Canary melon
- 2 oz. peeled and grated pumpkin

Directions:
1. Coat the grated pumpkin with honey.
2. Arrange the pumpkin, melon, apples and pumpkin seeds in a salad bowl.
3. Sprinkle with lemon juice.

Nutritional Information:
Calories: 213, Fat:6.5 g, Carbs:13 g, Protein:5 g, Sugars:1 g, Sodium:381 mg

Tuna Caprese Salad

Prep time: 10 mins | Servings: 2

Ingredients:
- 2 thinly sliced Roma tomatoes
- 2 tsps. balsamic vinegar
- 2 oz. cubed fresh mozzarella part-skim
- 8 large fresh basil leaves
- 1 tsp. olive oil
- 6 oz. fresh tuna steak
- Pepper
- 4 tsps. divided extra virgin olive oil

Directions:
1. On medium high fire, place a large skillet and heat 1 teaspoon olive oil.
2. Once hot, pan fry tuna for 3 minutes per side. Transfer to a plate with paper towel and dab dry. Place in ref to cool for at least an hour.
3. To assemble, layer tomatoes and tuna on a plate.
4. Season with pepper. Sprinkle with basil and mozzarella,
5. Drizzle balsamic vinegar and olive oil before serving.

Nutritional Information:
Calories: 267, Fat:14.6 g, Carbs:5.3 g, Protein:29.0 g, Sugars:2 g, Sodium:760 mg

Cabbage and Carrot Salad

Prep time: 5 mins | Servings: 4

Ingredients:
- 2 grated carrots
- 1 tbsp. lime juice
- 2 chopped shallots
- 1 tbsp. red vinegar
- ¼ tsp. black pepper
- 1 tbsp. olive oil
- 1 shredded big red cabbage head

Directions:
1. In a bowl, mix the cabbage with the shallots and the other ingredients, toss and serve as a salad.

Nutritional Information:
Calories: 106, Fat:3.8 g, Carbs:18 g, Protein:3.3 g, Sugars:1 g, Sodium:44 mg

Warm Asparagus Salad with Oranges

Prep time: 5 mins | Servings: 4

Ingredients:
- 1 lb. peeled and sliced fresh asparagus
- 2 tbsps. tomato basil seasoning blend
- 2 tbsps. olive oil
- 1 peeled and sectioned fresh orange

Directions:
1. Heat a 9 inch sauté pan to medium heat. Add olive oil.
2. When hot, add and toss asparagus. Cook 1 minute, tossing every 30 seconds.
3. Remove from heat, and toss with tomato basil seasoning blend and orange sections.

Nutritional Information:
Calories: 87.5, Fat:4.1 g, Carbs:8.1 g, Protein:5.1 g, Sugars:11 g, Sodium:10 mg

Chicken in Orange Sauce

Prep time: 10 mins | Servings: 4

Ingredients:
- ½ c. flour
- ¼ tsp. pepper
- 4 boneless and skinless chicken breasts
- ¼ tsp. salt
- 1 ½ c. orange juice
- 4 tbsps. margarine

Directions:
1. Rinse and pat dry the chicken. Cut into bite size pieces.
2. Place the flour in a shallow bowl.
3. In a large skillet, heat the margarine.
4. Dip the pieces of chicken in flour, fry in the margarine 4 - 6 minutes on each side, until golden brown.
5. Pour the orange juice over the chicken. Simmer until the orange juice is reduced, approximately 15 minutes.

Nutritional Information:
Calories: 160, Fat:18 g, Carbs:62 g, Protein:22 g, Sugars:19 g, Sodium:430 mg

Sweet Jicama Salad

Prep time: 12 mins | Servings: 1 - 2

Ingredients:
- 1 small fennel bulb
- ¼ tsp. salt
- ¼ lb. Jicama
- 1/8 tsp. fresh ground pepper
- ½ thinly sliced red onion
- Juice of 1 small tangerine
- 1 tbsp. chopped fennel leaves

Directions:
1. Peel and slice the Jicama into ¼ inch pieces.
2. Stem and core the fennel bulb, slice into thin half-moons.
3. In a large bowl, add the sliced Jicama and fennel. Squeeze the tangerine over the fennel and Jicama. Season with salt.
4. Garnish with black pepper and chopped fennel leaves. Serve immediately.

Nutritional Information:
Calories: 99, Fat:17 g, Carbs:35 g, Protein:45 g, Sugars:2 g, Sodium:405 mg

Heart Healthy Chicken Salad

Prep time: 10 mins | Servings: 5

Ingredients:
- ½ tsp. onion powder
- 1 tbsp. lemon juice
- 3 ¼ c. cooked, cubed, and skinless chicken breast
- 1 chopped lettuce head
- 3 tbsps. low-fat mayonnaise
- ¼ c. chopped celery

Directions:
1. Except for chicken and lettuce, combine all ingredients in a bowl and whisk well.
2. Add chicken and toss well to coat.
3. Evenly divide chopped lettuce in 5 bowls and top evenly with chicken salad.
4. Enjoy!

Nutritional Information:
Calories: 164, Fat:4.9 g, Carbs:1.9 g, Protein:28.3 g, Sugars:7 g, Sodium:179 mg

Cashews and Blueberries Salad

Prep time: 10 mins | Servings: 2

Ingredients:
- ¼ c. blueberries
- 1 peeled and sliced banana
- ¼ c. raw cashews
- 1 tsp. cinnamon powder
- 1 tbsp. almond butter

Directions:
1. In a bowl, combine the banana with cashews, blueberries, almond butter and cinnamon, toss and serve each day.
2. Enjoy!

Nutritional Information:
Calories: 120, Fat:0.3 g, Carbs:7 g, Protein:5 g, Sugars:5 g, Sodium:262 mg

Radish Salad

Prep time: 5 mins | Servings: 4

Ingredients:
- 1 lb. cubed radishes
- 1 c. pitted and halved black olives
- 2 tbsps. balsamic vinegar
- 2 tbsps. olive oil
- 2 green onions
- 1 tsp. chili powder
- ¼ tsp. black pepper

Directions:
1. In a large salad bowl, combine radishes with the onions and the other ingredients, toss and serve as a side dish.

Nutritional Information:
Calories: 123, Fat:10.8 g, Carbs:7 g, Protein:1.3 g, Sugars:1.7 g, Sodium:168 mg

Tarragon Tomatoes

Prep time: 5 mins | Servings: 4

Ingredients:
- 1 lb. sliced tomatoes
- 2 tbsps. chopped tarragon
- ¼ tsp. black pepper
- 1 ½ tbsps. olive oil
- 1 tbsp. grated lime zest
- 1 tbsp. lime juice

Directions:
1. In a bowl, combine the tomatoes with the other ingredients, toss and serve as a side salad.

Nutritional Information:
Calories: 170, Fat:4 g, Carbs:11.8 g, Protein:6 g, Sugars:9 g, Sodium:430 mg

Appendix 30 Day Meal Plan

	Breakfast	**Lunch**	**Dinner**	**Macros**
Day1	Egg Parsley Omelet	Beef with Cucumber Raita	Lamb Chops with Rosemary	Calorie:1874 Fat:174 Protein:58 Net Carb:19
Day2	Chocolate Covered Banana Quinoa	Pork and Cabbage Casserole	Authentic Pepper Steak	Calorie: 1892 Fat:176 Protein:62 Net Carb:25
Day3	Chocolate Covered Banana Quinoa	Curried Pork and Cabbage	Cane Wrapped Around In Prosciutto	Calorie:1976 Fat:164 Protein:88 Net Carb:37
Day4	Breakfast Apple and Raisin Oatmeal	Nutmeg Pork Chops	Beef Pot	Calorie:1994 Fat:186 Protein:44 Net Carb:36
Day5	Banana Nutty Oats	Butter and Dill Pork Chops	Lamb and Bok Choy Pan	Calorie:1731 Fat:163 Protein:27 Net Carb:39
Day6	Strawberry Chia Breakfast Pudding	Coconut Pork Chops	Beef & Vegetable Stir-Fry	Calorie:2000 Fat:168 Protein:99 Net Carb:23
Day7	Cherries Oatmeal	Pork with Chickpeas	Simple Veal Chops	Calorie:1946 Fat:162 Protein:89 Net Carb:33
Day8	Egg Spinach Breakfast Muffins	Pork and Mint Corn	Basil Tilapia	Calorie:1920 Fat:164 Protein:87 Net Carb:24
Day9	Breakfast Taco	Pork with Brussels Sprouts	Lemony Mussels	Calorie:1892 Fat:164 Protein:78 Net Carb:26
Day10	Cinnamon Walnut Breakfast Parfait	Pork with Beets	Hot Tuna Steak	Calorie:1821 Fat:161 Protein:79 Net Carb:14

Day11	Cinnamon Breakfast Quinoa	Pork and Green Onions Mix	"Marinated Fish Steaks	Calorie:1835 Fat:171 Protein:44 Net Carb:30
Day12	Granola Breakfast Pops	Pork and Carrots Soup	Baked Tomato Hake	Calorie:1912 Fat:168 Protein:76 Net Carb:24
Day13	Quinton Breakfast Bars	Pork with Herbs de Provence	Cheesy Tuna Pasta	Calorie:1869 Fat:161 Protein:75 Net Carb:30
Day14	Sweet Rosemary Oats	Sweet Rosemary Oats	Broiled White Sea Bass	Calorie:1784 Fat:164 Protein:52 Net Carb:25
Day15	Orange Juice Smoothie	Southwestern Salmon	Capelin Balls	Calorie:1844 Fat:160 Protein:78 Net Carb:23
Day16	Hearty Baby Carrots	Steamed Blue Crabs	Godly Garlic Butter Salmon Asparagus	Calorie:1890 Fat:168 Protein:52 Net Carb:45
Day17	Balsamic roast chicken	Spinach Spread	Falling "Off" The Bone Chicken	Calorie:1976 Fat:164 Protein:88 Net Carb:37
Day18	The Ultimate Faux-Tisserie Chicken	Slow-roast Chicken with Homemade Gravy	Turkey Pinwheels	Calorie:1895 Fat:163 Protcin:62 Net Carb:45
Day19	Chicken and Veggies	Hidden Valley Chicken Drummies	Chicken Divan	Calorie:1988 Fat:172 Protein:77 Net Carb:33
Day20	Chocolate Aquafaba Mousse	Minted Peas Feta Rice	Hearty Baby Carrots	Calorie:1994 Fat:186 Protein:44 Net Carb:36
Day21	Sensitive Steamed Artichokes	Salmon and Cauliflower Mix	Rhubarb and Strawberry Compote	Calorie1893 Fat:173 Protein:36 Net Carb:48

Day22	Easy Sautéed Fish Fillets	Creamy Salmon and Asparagus Mix	White sponge cake	Calorie:1731 Fat:163 Protein:27 Net Carb:39
Day23	Roasted asparagus	Rigatoni with broccoli	Rutabaga Puree	Calorie:1835 Fat:171 Protein:44 Net Carb:30
Day24	Hot Honey Porridge	Mango and Coconut Oatmeal	French Toast with Cinnamon Vanilla	Calorie:1946 Fat:162 Protein:89 Net Carb:33
Day25	Cheddar & Kale Frittata	Spinach Mushroom Omelette	Hearty Orange Peach Smoothie	Calorie1689 Fat:165 Protein:33 Net Carb:18
Day26	Breakfast Grains and Fruits	Spicy baked fish	Apple Cinnamon Overnight Oats	Calorie:1813 Fat:161 Protein:63 Net Carb:28
Day27	Breakfast Oatmeal in Slow Cooker	Steamed fish balls	Broiled White Sea Bass	Calorie:1892 Fat:164 Protein:78 Net Carb:26
Day28	Breakfast Banana Split	Curried Cauliflower Steaks with Red Rice	Dill Cabbage	Calorie:1929 Fat:161 Protein:97 Net Carb:23
Day29	Banana Bread	Parmesan and Chicken Spaghetti Squash	Oven-fried Chicken Breasts	Calorie:1912 Fat:168 Protein:76 Net Carb:24
Day30	Sunday Morning Waffles	Apricot Chicken	Rosemary Roasted Chicken	Calorie:1869 Fat:161 Protein:75 Net Carb:30

Conclusion

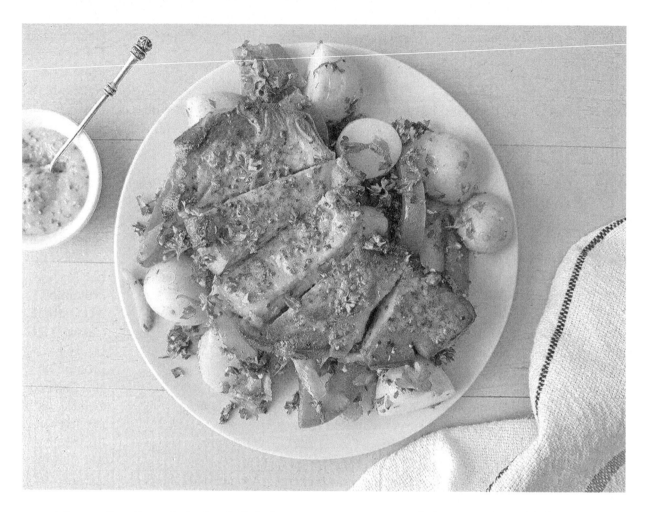

After reading through the book, it is important you get out and do as per the guideline. Choose a recipe, get the ingredients, throw them in your equipment and that's it. In just several minutes or a few hours, you will have a tasty and flavorful meal that will supply the body with healthy nutrients and will, at the same time, keep you away from sodium that can have many negative effects on your health. Choose wisely and use the food to your benefit.

Made in the USA
Monee, IL
02 April 2020